Tissue Engineering

Computational Methods in Applied Sciences

Volume 31

Series Editor

E. Oñate
International Center for Numerical Methods in Engineering (CIMNE)
Technical University of Catalonia (UPC)
Edificio C-1, Campus Norte UPC
Gran Capitán, s/n
08034 Barcelona, Spain
onate@cimne.upc.edu
url: http://www.cimne.com

For further volumes:
www.springer.com/series/6899

Paulo Rui Fernandes · Paulo Jorge Bártolo

Editors

Tissue Engineering

Computer Modeling, Biofabrication and Cell Behavior

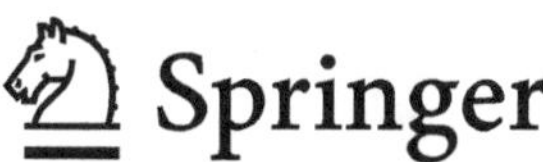 Springer

Editors
Paulo Rui Fernandes
Instituto Superior Tecnico
Mechanical Engineering Department
Technical University of Lisbon
Lisbon, Portugal

Paulo Jorge Bártolo
CDRSP – IP Leiria Portugal
Marinha Grande, Portugal

ISSN 1871-3033   Computational Methods in Applied Sciences
ISBN 978-94-007-7072-0   ISBN 978-94-007-7073-7 (eBook)
DOI 10.1007/978-94-007-7073-7
Springer Dordrecht Heidelberg New York London

Library of Congress Control Number: 2013945724

Printed on acid-free paper

Springer is part of Springer Science+Business Media (www.springer.com)

Preface

This book is a contribution for Tissue Engineering seen as multidisciplinary field involving scientists from different backgrounds like medicine, chemistry, material science, engineering and biology with a focus on the development of mathematical methods that are quite relevant to understand cell biology and human tissues as well to model, design and fabricate optimized and smart scaffolds.

The scientific interest of the computational mechanics community in Tissue Engineering, lead us to start a series of ECCOMAS Thematic Conferences on this field. It has been very successful event bringing together a considerable number of researchers from all over the world, representing several fields of study related to Tissue Engineering. As a consequence of these conferences a first book "Advances on Modelling in Tissue Engineering" was released in 2011. The present book, "Tissue Engineering: Computer Modeling, Biofabrication and Cell Behavior", consists of eight selected contributions of participants on the Second International Conference on Tissue Engineering, held in Lisbon in July 2011, covering these different aspects of Tissue Engineering.

The Editors are deeply grateful to the all the contributing authors. We would also like to thank the European Community on Computational Methods in Applied Sciences (ECCOMAS), the Portuguese Association of Theoretical Applied and Computational Mechanics (APMTAC), the Portuguese Foundation for Science and Technology (FCT), the Institute of Mechanical Engineering (IDMEC/IST) and the Centre for Rapid and Sustainable Product Development of the Polytechnic Institute of Leiria (CDRsp), for supporting the Conference.

Paulo Rui Fernandes
Paulo Jorge Bártolo

Contents

Stem Cell-Based Tissue Engineering for Bone Repair

Influence of Cell Communication and 3-D Cell-Matrix Environment

Swathi Damaraju and Neil A. Duncan

Abstract Culturing cells in 3D scaffolds can help model a physiological process. The property of the substrate used for such scaffolds has been shown to modify and determine stem cell lineage. Using this knowledge, *in-vitro* 3D stem cell culture models with *ex-vivo* bone tissue investigations can offer insight and inspiration for the development of novel therapies for bone defects. Although many different scaffolds have been created for bone tissue repair, *in situ* cell level mechanics are not always given consideration as the main design target. Overall, the ideal tissue engineering solution to bone regeneration would incorporate cells of osteogenic potential into a synthetic bone scaffold in order to reduce the need for external factors added such as drugs or growth factors. Attention to the mechanical aspects of the bone to be studied as well as the cells to be placed within the scaffold is fundamental. In this chapter, we will explore studies investigating the role of cell communication in bone mechanosensing, including the roles of different bone cells in the process of bone adaptation and repair, and the use of this knowledge in creating a novel tissue engineering strategy for the repair of acute bone defects.

1 The Skeleton

The human skeleton is a complex structure with critical structural, metabolic, and synthetic functions to perform. The ability of bone to coordinate these many functions in response to mechanical stimuli and biochemical factors, while retaining its mechanical properties, makes it a challenging structure to mimic in tissue engineering [1].

S. Damaraju (✉)
McCaig Institute for Bone and Joint Health, Faculty of Medicine, University of Calgary,
3280 Hospital Drive NW, Calgary, AB, T2N 4Z6, Canada
e-mail: sdamaraj@ucalgary.ca

N.A. Duncan
Departments of Civil Engineering and Surgery, Schulich School of Engineering,
University of Calgary, 2500 University Drive NW, Calgary, AB, T2N 1N4, Canada
e-mail: duncan@ucalgary.ca

P.R. Fernandes, P.J. Bártolo (eds.), *Tissue Engineering*,
Computational Methods in Applied Sciences 31, DOI 10.1007/978-94-007-7073-7_1,

The macro-scale structure of bone enables it to protect the internal organs, provide a support frame for the body, allow movement through the interactions with muscles, as well as produce blood cells. In addition to these functions, the micro-scale properties of bone allow it to regulate mineral storage, fat storage, and phosphate metabolism [1].

The mechanical properties and biological functions of bone are derived from the cells, water, and the extracellular matrix proteins—chiefly, type-I collagen [1]. The mineral component of the extracellular matrix, a form of calcium phosphate called hydroxyapatite, gives bone its hardness, while type-I collagen gives bone its flexibility. The ability of bone to remodel and repair itself is due to the coordinated function of cells, along with the presence of bone marrow. Bone marrow contains hematopoietic and non-hematopoietic stem cells from which osteoclasts and osteoblasts respectively originate [1].

Engineering scaffolds that can incorporate these components to augment bone healing is a key research area in bone tissue regeneration. Strategies that promote endogenous or synthetic repair mechanisms have been investigated. It is currently unknown which mechanism is optimal for engineered bone regeneration, although a design mimicking endogenous repair seems to be the most promising [2].

2 Bone Formation and Healing

2.1 Fracture Healing

Fracture healing in long bones involves a series of events beginning with inflammation, followed by formation of a hematoma (clot) surrounded by the periosteal layer of bone. The repair process of the fracture site is organized by the structure of the hematoma [3]. The structure of the hematoma provides a scaffold in which rapid cell division can occur [3]. Within this scaffold, the possible sources of the osteogenic cells involved in enabling fracture repair have been debated. One theory suggests that the repair tissue arises from cells that are predetermined to differentiate into bone, while the second theory asserts that the repair tissue is formed from the activity of uncommitted cells that develop osteogenic potential given certain environmental stimuli, a process termed "osteogenic induction" [3].

The first theory described above likely refers to mesenchymal stem cells that are predetermined to an osteogenic fate, while the second theory describes cell types that are similar to pluripotent embryonic stem cells [3, 4]. With regards to the first theory, it is well known that during bone formation, osteoblasts are recruited from mesenchymal stem cells in the bone marrow, while osteoclasts are formed from hematopoietic stem cells predetermined to a monocyte lineage [3]. It has also been determined that the bone marrow stroma contains fibroblast-like stem cells that also possess osteogenic potential [4]. These cells are referred to as bone marrow stromal cells (BMSC), though their exact location *in-vivo* is yet to be determined [4].

Both mesenchymal and embryonic stem cells have been investigated as osteogenic sources for stem cell repair of bone defects. The findings from these studies will be outlined further in this chapter.

2.2 Clinical Therapies for Fracture Repair

Although there are many treatment options for bone repair, the extent and quality of repair that occurs from these strategies is inconsistent. Physiological impairment of fracture healing can be caused by pathologies such as osteoporosis, osteogenesis imperfecta, or defects in the mechanical stability or vascular supply of the bone at the time of fracture [5]. In all of these cases, nonunion fractures are likely to develop.

> Nonunions are fractures that fail to heal naturally 6–8 months after the time of fracture. In the human population, approximately 10 % of fractures fail to heal naturally [5]. Risk factors for nonunions include smoking, aging, anemia, diabetes, use of anti-inflammatory drugs, infection, and lack of calcium and vitamin D in the diet. The main symptom of a nonunion is persistent pain at the breakage site, and can be conclusively diagnosed with x-ray, magnetic resonance, or computed tomography imaging [5].

Currently, nonsurgical treatment of nonunions involves the application of a bone stimulator. The stimulator uses ultrasonic or electromagnetic waves to stimulate healing [5, 6]. However, the patient must be diligent in wearing the external device for 20 minutes to 2 hours every day. Because of this, the rate and quality of fracture healing is highly dependent on consistency of use [6].

Surgical treatments of nonunions include bone grafts, internal fixation, and external fixation [7, 8]. For bone grafting procedures, the bone for the graft is usually taken from the rim of the pelvis or iliac crest of the patient [8]. However, these procedures can be very painful and have low bone yield. As well, the use of bone grafts alone does not provide any initial stability to the defect [8].

In defects where mechanical stability is required, internal or external fixation is used [7, 8]. For internal fixation, metal plates and screws are attached to the outside of the bone, or rods are placed inside the bone canal to confer additional mechanical stability to the fracture [8]. This type of fixation can also be combined with bone grafts.

External fixation involves a rigid frame positioned outside of the defective limb that is attached to the internal bone by pins or wires [8]. Distraction osteogenesis (also called the Ilizarov method) can be used with external fixation to stretch the developing callus between the fractured segments of the bone [8]. Inducing new bone growth by this method is achieved by creating a uniform rate of mechanical strain, which is suggested to increase the activity of osteoprogenitor cells, and thus increase the production and mineralization of the extracellular matrix leading to new bone formation [7, 8].

Increased mechanical stability with internal or external fixation promotes fracture healing and angiogenesis [4, 8]. However, the differentiation of osteoprogenitor cells within a bone defect depends on the type of mechanical load applied [4]. Depending on the size of the defect and amount of callus formation, the extent of osteogenic differentiation may be supported or restricted by stabilizing the fracture [4]. For example, it has been demonstrated that tensile strain in a fracture gap causes the callus to cleave, and subsequently promotes fibrocartilage formation instead of bone [4]. Therefore, despite the beneficial effects of current surgical treatments for nonunions, further study of the effect of mechanical stability on a fracture would provide a greater understanding of what factors are necessary for normal bone healing, the coordinated actions of the cells involved, and the potential tissue engineering strategies that could be designed from this knowledge.

3 Structures for Cell Communication

It has been suggested that intercellular signaling plays a crucial role in the establishment of cooperative functioning in cell populations [11]. Information required for development and proper functioning of cells may be transferred through direct cell-cell contacts, such as gap junctions, cadherins, integrins, and cytoplasmic bridges, or through ligand-receptor mechanisms at the cell surface. In bone, it has been shown that gap junctions, cadherins, and integrins are highly involved in osteoblast, osteoclast, and osteocyte activity [9].

3.1 Gap Junctions in Bone Cells

Gap junction communication is hypothesized to be critical in the coordination of bone remodeling [10–12]. The cells in bone, namely, osteoblasts, and osteocytes, have been shown to express connexin 43, 45, and 46, while osteoclasts and chondrocytes in bone have been shown to primarily express connexin 43 [10]. Gap junctions are membrane channels that are formed by the docking of two hemichannels on adjacent cells. The gap junctional hemichannel, also called a connexon, is formed by a hexameric arrangement of proteins termed connexins [10]. Each connexin protein is composed of four membrane spanning domains consisting of two small extracellular loops, an intracellular loop, and intracellular amino and carboxyl ends [11]. More than 17 connexin genes have been identified in mice, and more than 20 in humans [10, 11]. In the human body, connexins are present in a variety of cell types, providing evidence for their importance in a host of organ and cell functions.

Gap junctions allow the diffusion of ions, metabolites, and signaling molecules between adjacent cells [11]. Depending on the connexin gene that is expressed, the resulting gap junction channel formed will possess specific charge and size permeability [10]. The most abundant connexin in bone is connexin 43 [10, 11].

A gap junction channel formed from connexin 43 proteins allows molecules less than 1.2 kDa in molecular mass to pass through, with a preference for negatively charged molecules, such as intracellular calcium, cyclic adenosine monophosphate (cAMP), and adenosine triphosphate (ATP) [10]. Connexin proteins can also form as homomeric or heteromeric connexons. For example, connexin 43 and 45 are able to assemble into a hemichannel composed of both proteins. This combination of two different connexin proteins results in a channel with differences in the channel's biochemical and electrical properties [10]. It has been shown that connexin hemichannels regulate the release of ATP and prostaglandin E2 in response to mechanical stimulation [10, 11].

As mentioned above, gap junctions are present in many different tissues. In addition to being present in fully differentiated organs, gap junctions are also critically involved in many phases of embryonic development and patterning, including skeletal development [10, 12]. Bone formation is orchestrated by two mechanisms: intramembranous and endochondral ossification. The majority of bones are formed via endochondral ossification, in which a cartilaginous template is formed by chondrocytes prior to vascularization and mineralization by osteoblasts [12]. In intramembranous ossification, mesenchyme condensations of cells differentiate into osteoblasts that mineralize the extracellular matrix in the absence of a cartilaginous precursor [12]. In the process of mineralization, some osteoblasts get trapped within the unmineralized matrix (called the osteoid) and become osteocytes that connect to one another via gap junctions at the ends of their long cell processes. The gap junctions between osteocytes are regulated by parathyroid hormone and pH [10–12]. It has been shown that a low pH environment causes uncoupling of gap junctions and reduces the expression of connexin 43 in osteocytes [11]. As well, administration of parathyroid hormone to osteocytes has been shown to cause increased gap junction activity, measured by fluorescence recovery after photobleaching (FRAP) [13]. Osteoblasts on the surface of bone are also connected via gap junctions.

3.1.1 Gap Junctions in Osteoblasts

The gap junctions present between osteoblasts on the bone surface are suggested to play a role in regulating bone remodeling [12]. *In-vitro* experiments have shown that during osteoblast differentiation, connexin 43 expression increased, and as a result, the amount of gap junction-mediated communication increased as well [10, 12]. Furthermore, inhibition of these connexin 43 gap junctions resulted in impaired osteoblast differentiation, a reduced ability of the cells to mineralize the extracellular matrix, and reduced expression of osteoblastic genes, specifically collagen I and osteocalcin [10, 12]. Not only was osteoblast differentiation impaired, but the use of inhibitors such as 18-α-glycyrrhetinic acid caused trans-differentiation of cells into adipocytes [10]. Extensive study of connexin 43 has revealed that a specific DNA binding domain within the protein confers connexin sensitivity to both the osteocalcin and collagen I promoters by binding specific transcription factors [12]. Therefore, it is believed that connexin 43 mediated communication affects osteoblast gene expression by interfering with specific signaling molecules that are activated via extracellular stimuli [12]. Connexin-containing gap junctions thus control the propagation of signals by either permitting or restricting the passage of secondary messengers used in important signaling pathways. Gap junction-mediated control of signaling molecules has been shown in the RANKL pathway, which controls osteoclastogenesis [14].

Further studies demonstrating the importance of these junctions *in-vivo* was established through human and mouse genetic experiments. Connexin 43 knockout mice showed phenotypes with reduced mineralization of craniofacial bones and delayed ossification in the long bones of the skeleton [12, 15]. This phenotype resembled a human genetic defect in connexin 43, that leads to human oculodentodigital dysplasia (ODDD). The link between the phenotype of the knockout mouse to the appearance of the human disease is the strongest evidence for the critical role connexin 43 plays in skeletal function and development [12, 15].

3.1.2 Gap Junctions in Osteocytes

Gap junctions have also been implicated in playing a role in the mechanosensing ability of bone [12, 15]. It is generally agreed that deformation of the bone matrix by physical load generates an array of biophysical signals that affects bone cell activity and differentiation [18]. In this response, fluid flow is thought to represent the primary biophysical signal in bone mechanotransduction [12, 15]. For example, it has been shown that osteoblasts and osteocytes remodel their connexin 43 and 45 gap junctions in response to fluid shear stress [12, 15]. At low shear stress, osteoblasts and osteocytes increased connexin 43 expression, while decreasing connexin 43 expression at high shear stress [10, 12]. It has also been shown that connexin 43 channels and hemichannels are active in osteocytes, and that these junctions mediate fluid flow-induced prostaglandin and ATP release [10, 12]. The precise role of connexins in mechanically-induced fluid flow release from osteocytes has been difficult to determine. This is primarily due to the fact that current methods of measurement are not sensitive enough to distinguish between diffusion of a molecule through a gap junction, and other methods of transport, such as exocytosis [10, 12].

Of all the cells present in bone, osteocytes seem to be the best candidate to be mechanoreceptors within the bone [10, 12]. Osteocytes have cell processes that pass through channels in the bone called canaliculi, and are connected to each other via gap junctions [11, 17]. The role of gap junctions in bone mechanotransduction has been proposed because of their ability to propagate intracellular signals produced under mechanical strain. For example, prostaglandin E2 is an intracellular signal which is dependent on mechanically-induced gap junction activity [11]. It has been shown that fluid flow causes upregulation of gap junction activity by the ERK1/2 MAP-kinase pathway [11]. This stimulates connexin 43 expression, and release of prostaglandin E2. Other pathways controlling the release of intracellular signals such as ATP and cAMP behave similarly when subjected to mechanical stimulation.

Only a few studies have been performed that investigate the expression and regulation of connexin 43 under the influence of mechanical stimulation [11, 16, 17]. As well, few studies have been performed to investigate the downstream physiological response due to mechanotransduction of a signal from osteocytes to osteoblasts [11, 12]. It is believed that calcium signaling plays a role in bone mechanotransduction. Gap junctions in the osteocytic network are capable of propagating calcium waves between cells [15, 18]. When one cell is mechanically stimulated, a wave of calcium signals is created and propagated between adjacent cells [18]. It is thought this gap junction mode of wave propagation is carried out through intercellular diffusion of secondary messengers that control calcium release [18]. Intercellular propagation of calcium can also be caused by hormones and growth factors [11]. The propagation of calcium waves through the osteocytic network causes activation of the ERK signaling pathway, and thus promotes production of prostaglandin E2 [11]. It has been demonstrated that in osteoblasts, increased intracellular levels of calcium ion causes uncoupling of cells. However, upon an increase in extracellular calcium ion influx, the subsequent increase in intracellular calcium ion concentration is transmitted through connexin-43 gap junctions [11]. It is hypothesized that the coordinated propagation of calcium ion waves by gap junctions provides a mechanism for organizing large populations of osteocytes within bone to be able to respond in a coordinated manner [11].

The differential effect of mechanics on osteocytes versus osteoblasts has been elucidated. *In-vitro* studies performed in a rat tooth model showed increased connexin 43 expression in osteoclasts under compression, and in osteoblasts and osteocytes under tension [11, 16], suggesting connexin 43 expression is highly sensitive to mechanical loading. Mechanical loading has also been shown *in-vitro* to be essential for phosphorylation of connexin 43, thereby enabling functional formation of gap junction channels in osteoblast cells [11, 16, 17]. In addition to these studies, a novel *in-vitro* system was used to subject osteocytes to fluid flow, while osteoblasts were left unloaded [19]. When osteocytes were exposed to fluid flow, alkaline phosphatase activity (an important factor for mineralization of the extracellular matrix) increased in osteoblasts [18, 19]. Conversely, when osteoblasts were subjected to fluid flow, no such effect was observed [19]. In addition to this, inhibition of the connexin 43 gap junctions resulted in a lack of propagation of mechanical signal to the osteoblasts via the osteocytic network [19]. This evidence suggests that direct physical contact between osteocytes and osteoblasts is necessary for osteoblast response to physical signals.

To date, it is believed that calcium, prostaglandin E2, and cAMP are a few of the signals necessary to convey mechanical signals to osteocytes and the extracellular matrix as part of the remodeling process of bone [11, 17]. Deformation of the bone matrix by mechanical stimuli produces these biophysical signals that affects bone cell activity and differentiation [15, 18]. This in turn contributes to the anabolic response to mechanical load. However further investigation is required to determine the precise roles of these molecules, and any addition molecules that could be involved.

3.1.3 Gap Junctions in Osteoclasts

Connexin 43 has also been implicated to play a role in osteoclast formation [11, 15]. Osteoclasts are bone cells responsible for breaking down and resorbing bone, as part of the natural remodeling and turnover characteristic of bone tissue [11]. Gap junctions have been shown to play an important role in enabling fusion of osteoclast precursors in order to form functional multinucleated mature osteoclasts [11, 15]. Multiple studies using gap junction inhibitors have shown that gap junction intercellular communication is essential for osteoclast formation and survival [11, 12, 15], and is thus essential for bone remodeling to occur.

The differentiation and activation of osteoclasts is regulated by RANKL (receptor activator of NF-κB ligand) signaling [14]. RANK receptors are found on osteoblasts [14]. Binding of RANK ligand to RANK receptors on osteoblasts stimulates osteoclast differentiation and activation. The role of gap junctions in the RANKL control of osteoclastogenesis has been investigated. In this study, carbenoxolone, a gap junction inhibitor, was applied to mouse bone marrow cells. This treatment caused inhibition of RANKL-mediated osteoclast activation in the cultures [14]. Therefore, the investigators of this study suggested that gap junction mediated diffusion of a critical signaling molecule had downstream effects on RANKL signaling and thus inhibited osteoclast differentiation and activation [14]. The exact mechanism of this effect is yet to be determined.

3.1.4 Other Functions of Gap Junctions in Bone

Gap junctions also regulate apoptosis [18]. This function is due to the formation of gap junction hemichannels activating a signaling cascade that leads to inhibition of apoptosis [18].

3.2 Cadherins in Bone

Cadherins are part of a family of adherens junctions that allow homophilic, calcium-dependent intercellular adhesion [12, 20, 21]. Cadherins are composed of 30 single chain integral membrane lycoproteins that are approximately 120 kDa in size [12].

Cadherin junctions consist of a long N-terminal extracellular domain, a transmembrane domain, and a small intracellular C-terminal [18]. Many different tissues express multiple cadherins.

> In bone, osteogenic cells during differentiation express a variety of cadherins. R-cadherin/cadherin-4 is downregulated as differentiation progresses, while cadherin-11 (also known as osteoblast-cadherin, or OB-Cad) is upregulated [12]. N-cadherin is the most abundant cadherin, as it is present throughout osteogenic differentiation [15, 18].

In-vitro studies of bone have shown that cultured osteoblasts also express N-cadherin and cadherin-11 [20, 21]. Using various inhibitors of these cadherins, researchers have shown that blocking cadherin expression in osteoblast lineage cells impairs differentiation into osteoblasts [20, 21], thereby demonstrating the necessity for cadherins in full osteoblast phenotype development [12]. In addition to *in-vitro* approaches, isolating the function of cadherins in bone requires *in-vivo* study. Experiments involving genetic deletion of the N-cadherin gene in mice has been shown to lead to an embryonic lethal product [12, 21]. However, heterozygous N-cad mutants were shown to have normal bone density with an osteoblast abnormality identified [12]. Homozygous cadherin-11 deficient animals have been shown to develop a phenotype that appears normal at birth, but then progresses to defects in the calcification of cranial sutures, and osteopenia (a condition where the bone mineral density is low) in trabecular bone, both of which are pathologies linked to a defect in the functionality of osteoblasts [12, 21]. Extensive work on the role of OB-Cad in bone has shown that this protein is not only responsible for osteoblast differentiation and function, but also is involved in bone marrow cell lineage determination and signaling [20, 21]. Cadherins have also been shown to be involved in osteogenic commitment of mesenchymal stem cells, primarily through β-catenin signaling [12].

Cadherins have also been implicated to be important for mechanotransduction [22]. *In-vitro* experiments involving plating surfaces with cadherin extracellular domains caused spreading and clustering of cells, as well as organization of cadherins into streaks on the surface [22, 23]. Moreover, it was demonstrated that cells with N-cadherin complexes exerted traction forces on the surface which they were on [22, 24]. Studies of the cadherin-mediated mechanotransduction in bone still need to be investigated, however studies in more specialized systems have been examined. For example, the response of the villi on inner ear hair cells to sound waves is mediated by a conformational change in cadherin structure that transmits the sound wave force to stretch-activated channels [22]. These channels then open, allowing conductance to occur.

Therefore, since these cell junctions are integral in both embryonic and mesenchymal stem cell differentiation, and seem to play a role in mechanotransduction, understanding how they are regulated and the impact of their presence on cell surface adhesion will help us understand the mechanisms by which stem cells are guided to different lineages [12, 21]. The knowledge gained from this and from further investigation of cadherins and the role of mechanical stimulation in the regulation of osteoblast cadherin-mediated bone differentiation will contribute to the potential for therapies targeted towards osteogenesis.

3.3 Integrins in Bone

Integrins are another type of adhesion receptor that regulate cell-cell adhesion, and cell-matrix interactions [20, 27]. Integrins are heterodimeric membrane glycoproteins, consisting of an α and β subunit, each with a large extracellular domain and a short cytoplasmic domain [29].

> To date, although there are a variety of integrins, the focus has been on the $\alpha v\beta 3$ integrin which is highly expressed in osteoclasts [28, 29]. In fact, this integrin has been shown to be essential for osteoclasts to maintain their ability to resorb bone [29]. In order for osteoclasts to resorb bone as part of the remodeling process of bone adaptation and repair, integrins are used to adhere to the extracellular matrix proteins on the bone surface [20, 27].

The first demonstration that $\alpha v\beta 3$ integrins are important in regulating osteoclast function was shown with an antibody raised against osteoclasts, which consequently inhibited bone resorption *in-vitro* [11, 28, 29]. Interfering with this integrin through the use of RGD-containing peptides also led to inhibition of bone resorption both *in-vitro* and *in-vivo* [28, 29]. The mechanism through which $\alpha v\beta 3$ integrin acts in osteoclasts is not yet understood. Many *in-vitro* investigations have shown that this integrin is necessary for many initial adhesion events in osteoclasts, with the addition of $\alpha v\beta 3$ integrin blockers resulting in total inhibition of osteoclast adhesion, or retraction of osteoclasts in bone [29]. It is therefore hypothesized that $\alpha v\beta 3$ integrin enables cell adhesion, and plays a regulatory role in osteoclast migration [29]. Osteoclast migration is known to be necessary for effective bone resorption by osteoclasts, and therefore $\alpha v\beta 3$ integrin is thought to also mediate cell migration in osteoclasts [28, 29]. Integrins are regulated by extracellular factors that interact with the external domain of the integrin structure, thus stimulating downstream signaling [29]. Osteoclasts highly express a factor called c-Src, whose absence in bone causes complete inhibition of bone resorption *in-vivo* without affecting osteoclast cell number [28, 29]. In addition to this molecule, a cytokine known as interleukin-1 (IL-1) interacts with $\alpha v\beta 3$ signaling to stimulate *in-vitro* and *in-vivo* bone resorption [29]. Since $\alpha v\beta 3$ integrin is capable of transmitting signals to regulate osteoclasts, modifying this integrin's activity can be achieved by differing expression levels at the cell surface, levels of intracellular signals used to activate integrin signaling, and levels of cytokines, growth factors, and other molecules that interact with the components of this integrin [29].

Integrin signaling has been shown to play a role in mechanotransduction [22]. It has been shown that subjecting integrins to tension causes fast recruitment of adhesion molecules such as vinculin and zyxin [22]. It was also demonstrated that tension causes a conformation change in the integrin structure which enables them to bind to specific extracellular matrix proteins [22]. Further studies have demonstrated that strain applied to adherent cells caused activation of c-Src, a factor necessary for osteoclast function [22]. In bone, when a component of integrin signaling known as focal adhesion kinase (FAK) was inhibited, the remodeling response of osteoblasts and osteoclasts was absent [25]. As well, the ERK 1/2 pathway was found to be mediated by integrin signaling, and more importantly, play a role in the mechanotransduction mechanism behind distraction osteogenesis [26]. The specific mechanisms underlying the above responses of integrins to mechanical stimulation are yet to be identified. It is believed that after loading is applied, the initial conformational change in integrin structure is the critical step to initiate a response.

Significant evidence shows $\alpha v \beta 3$ integrin to be essential in osteoclast bone resorption, and through modifications of $\alpha v \beta 3$ integrin activity, this integrin is now viewed as a potential target in diseases such as osteoporosis and rheumatoid arthritis [28, 29]. Therapeutic approaches targeted towards integrin inhibition for pathologies such as osteoporosis could be effective, but further investigation into the role of mechanical stimulation on the activity of $\alpha v \beta 3$ integrin is necessary.

3.4 Conclusions

Increased knowledge of intercellular and cell-matrix structures may be used to determine a more detailed understanding of the role of gap junctions, cadherins, and integrins in regulating the adaptation and remodeling of bone in response to mechanical stimulation. In order to identify an engineered strategy for bone repair, the role and level of cell communication during bone healing needs further investigation.

4 Tissue Engineering for Bone Regeneration

As described at the beginning of this chapter, bone is a complex tissue that is responsible for supporting the body, protecting the organs, and forming blood cells. In addition, the development of bone involves two intricate mechanisms, intramembranous and endochondral ossification, along with a well vascularized environment. Since bone formation is so complex, defects in the physiological functioning of bone cells can occur in addition to the mechanically caused defects (nonunions) [4]. Both types of defects present a major challenge for bone repair. As mentioned earlier, because of the disadvantages of bone grafting procedures, the search for an efficient biocompatible bone transplant material for mechanical and physiological defects is of utmost importance. In fact, of the many available synthetic bone substitutes used clinically today, although all are successful in enabling repair in a laboratory setting, none to date are consistent enough in promoting bone repair in populations of patients clinically [4].

There are many tissue engineering strategies that have been developed for bone regeneration, but a design that can fulfill all mechanical and biological requirements of a bone substitute is yet to be developed [4]. For this purpose, choosing the right biomaterial is crucial in developing functional tissue-engineered organs. It is thought that the ideal bone biomaterial would possess a biodegradable capacity, with a structure that is well vascularized, and that integrates with host cells to stimulate their function, or, as a scaffold seeded with cells, function on its own to form bone [4]. Therefore, a scaffold material that enables cell communication, cell adherence, as well as cell maintenance is critical. For this reason, an understanding of gap junctions, cadherins, and integrins will be paramount to developing this design.

Some tissue engineering strategies involve injection or molding of biodegradable materials into tissues [4]. These strategies often involve modifying known cells, polymers, and mechanics of already developed geometric scaffolds. For these strategies to be successful, the most important aspect of their design is that the injected or shaped scaffold placed within the tissue must be able to restore the form and function of the tissue to its original state [4]. Ideally, the scaffold material will degrade as form and function returns to the tissue, creating a system that follows "programmed decomposition" [4].

For bone tissue engineering, one of the main challenges in creating such a scaffold is that the mechanical characteristics of the scaffold will change as it degrades and allows the perfusion of nutrients and solutes [30, 31, 33, 34]. Therefore the foundation of this design rests on the need for increased bone formation during repair to compensate and increase the mechanical strength of the defect as the mechanical properties of the scaffold decrease [30, 33, 34]. The ability of bone to grow into the scaffold is also necessary [30]. Ideally, the bone remodeling occurring within the scaffold would lead to complete healing of the bone defect [30, 32, 35].

By using molecules and materials endogenous to the human body, an optimal engineering design for a scaffold can be determined to enhance the activity of the surrounding cells in the tissue [4]. With the addition of cells to the scaffold itself, this design may be able to expedite the healing process by initiating healing within the scaffold itself rather than at its periphery. For this reason, combinations of cell and biomaterial-based scaffolds are promising strategies that are investigated in tissue engineering research today. However, many details on the optimal biomaterial-cell combination still need to be determined through extensive research before reaching a clinical stage [4]. Specifically, the effect of biomechanics on cells within the scaffold as well as the scaffold itself needs to be taken into account [30]. In addition to adding growth factors and choosing materials to promote bone growth, the cells themselves need to be controlled through mechanical loading, both in regulation of differentiation and proliferation into bone [30, 32, 35].

4.1 Mechanical Considerations for Bone Regeneration

Biomechanical studies in the past have focused on orthopedic implants [30]. The knowledge acquired from these studies can be applied to bone tissue engineering, especially the mechanical properties and interface conditions required for the scaffold to promote bone regeneration *in-vivo* [30, 31, 35]. Different tissue engineering applications of scaffolds require different biomechanical properties. For bone repair, such as in tibial defects, the demands of the created scaffold for a load-bearing tissue are highest [30–32].

Therefore, for bone applications, tissue engineering approaches aim to create scaffolds in such a way that they can function immediately upon insertion into the defect [30–32, 35]. Bone mechanics play an important role in determining the mechanical properties needed for a scaffold. The scaffold created must be able to withstand *in-vivo* forces transmitted by the tissue as well as normal loading conditions post-surgery [30, 31]. The mechanical properties of the bone to be formed within the scaffold need to be defined, as well as the permeability to fluid flow in order to mimic *in-vivo* properties and fluid flow conditions [30, 32]. In addition to mimicking bone mechanical properties, the loading conditions for the scaffold need to be defined [30]. In the case of tibial repairs, many investigators create a scaffold reinforced with calcium phosphate particles [30, 33]. However, many different scaffolds have been created for bone tissue repair, and few have taken the role of mechanical stimulation in bone repair into consideration as the main scaffold design target [30, 32, 33]. To this end, many studies have investigated the development of a biodegradable, or porous scaffold, that can transport solutes, or in some designs, degrades as repair of the bone defect progresses [30, 31, 35]. In general, it is agreed upon that scaffolds that allow tissue growth, nutrient diffusion, and vascularization are optimal for bone repair [30–32, 34]. For the most part, the present knowledge gained on mechanotransduction has been used for the development of bioreactors to optimize *in-vitro* bone formation in scaffolds [30, 32, 33]. The *in-vitro* bioreactor approach to create functional bone has not yet been fully successful [30]. Problems arise due to lack of consistency in the derived tissue, as well as determining the optimal perfusion velocities without subjecting the cells to a detrimental shear stress [30]. Given the challenges in engineering bone-promoting bioreactors, alternative methods using the bone surrounding a large bone defect as the so called "bioreactor" may be more successful in producing an engineered bone construct [30, 35]. This concept has been demonstrated in a rabbit model where an artificial space between the tibia and the periosteum was created and filled with a hydrogel, thereby mimicking an *in-vivo* bioreactor. The "bioreactor" from this study resulted in new bone formation with mechanical properties similar to that of native bone [30, 35].

Therefore, it may be that the best environment for bone scaffolds are the native bone itself, with the idea that a scaffold could mature into normal bone as long as an adequate environment is provided [30, 31, 33–35]. Overall, an approach to bone regeneration would incorporate osteogenic cells into a bone scaffold that, ideally, reduces the need for external factors (such as drugs or growth factors) to be added [30]. Mechanical aspects of native bone as well as the cells to be inserted within the scaffold are therefore fundamental to define in order to successfully produce a tissue engineering solution to large bone defects [30].

4.2 Conclusions

From the evidence presented above, it appears that the ideal bone scaffold must possess three characteristics: (1) the correct geometry to define and maintain an anatomic space in which it is placed, (2) provide temporary load-bearing within a defect, and (3) enhance the regenerative capacity of the cells placed within the defect or enhance the repair capacity of the tissue around the defect [4]. For load-bearing purposes, achieving stiffness and strength equivalent to that in bone requires minimally porous scaffolds [4]. However, if enhanced delivery of biofactors or cells need to be placed within the scaffold, then this requires a more highly connected porous scaffold to allow cell migration and vascularization within the scaffold [4]. Thus, experimentation with different scaffold materials, porosities, and cell densities needs to occur before a scaffold can be developed that matches complex anatomic defects, while providing biological and mechanical support.

5 Synthetic Scaffolds

A variety of synthetic polymers have been examined for bone tissue engineering. Polymers have been investigated because the rate of degradation and mechanical properties of the polymers can be controlled, as opposed to using natural compounds that are biological in origin [4]. Of the many available degradable polymers, aliphatic polyesters are the most prominently used in tissue engineering strategies, since the chemistry of these polymers renders them capable of interacting in hydrolytic and enzymatic reactions that produces hydroxyacids [4]. A common polymer that belongs to the polyester family is PLLA, which is a poly(-hydroxy acid). However, scaffolds with PLLA have been shown to be hydrophobic, making them difficult to incorporate into the body, as well as unreactive, making it difficult to attach drugs or cells to enhance its intended medical action [4]. For this reason, biodegradable copolymers have been investigated as potential bone biomaterials. Copolymers offer the advantage of being able to modulate the chemical and mechanical properties of the scaffold by merely adjusting the ratio of the polymers involved [4].

Table 1 Mechanical properties of polymer-based scaffolds [37, 39, 40]

Polymer	Tensile strength (MPa)	Modulus (GPa)
PLLA	10–60	0.35–2.8
PLLA-poly(ethylene glycol)	7–36	0.15-0.44
poly(lactide-co-glycolide)	20–40	2.7
poly(1,5-dioxepan-2-one)	27–39	0.16

> Several copolymers of relevance to bone regeneration are poly(1,5-dioxepan), PLLA-poly(ethylene glycol), and poly(lactide-co-glycolide).

Poly(lactide-co-glycolide) has been shown to induce bone regeneration, but its poor mechanical properties makes it an ineffective material for bone scaffolds [4]. The PLLA-poly(ethylene glycol) copolymer is still being investigated. Modulating both components causes changes in the crystallinity of the scaffold, and it is believed that this can be optimized to produce a structure that is similar to the crystalline structure of bone extracellular matrix, while also being hydrophilic, allowing the attachment of cells and drugs to the scaffold [4, 36]. Finally, poly(1,5-dioxepan) is a polymer that is normally soft, giving it good elastic and degradation properties, but when copolymerized with lactide, results in a rigid crystalline structure. Copolymerization with lactide improves the mechanical properties of the structure and changes the hydrophilic nature of the scaffold as well [4, 37, 38]. Experiments using poly(1,5-dioxepan-2-one) in different copolymer ratios in *in-vitro* cell culture have shown that this polymer could be used as a scaffold for bone tissue engineering [4]. Table 1 shows the mechanical properties of these polymer based scaffolds.

Therefore, as opposed to using one polymer to make up a scaffold, copolymerization allows the creation of multiple reactive sites, with the potential for modulating the chemical and mechanical properties of the scaffold depending on what medical application is desired.

Although copolymerization allows the controlled modification of scaffold properties, several adverse effects of using synthetic polymers have been demonstrated after implantation. The most relevant of these effects is the interaction of the polymers with the host's immune system. Implantation of the polymers described above have caused immune reactions in some patients ranging from the release of large numbers of white blood cells, to resorption of the original tissue [4, 41]. Therefore, greater understanding of the relationship between biocompatibility of a material before implantation, and its mechanical adaptation when placed inside the body needs to be further investigated. Proper sterilization of the material without compromising biomechanical stability, in addition to possessing properties that inhibits fibrotic tissue formation and immune reaction will help to create a synthetic biomaterial that can be used safely for degradable tissue engineering scaffolds in bone [4, 41].

5.1 Conclusions

The use of synthetic materials for scaffolds allows the manipulation of chemical properties by copolymerization, mechanical properties by changing the ratio of chemical polymers involved, as well as introducing different architectural designs (connected pores in triangles, pentagons, and honeycombs) to the scaffold. In the creation of such scaffolds, controlling the degradable nature of the biomaterial is crucial [4, 41]. Degradability ultimately relies on the chemical structure, architecture, and morphology of the scaffold, so a synthetic material that contains copolymers associated with crystalline materials are the most promising [4]. With these approaches and considerations, synthetic bone scaffolds carry enormous potential and thorough investigation into their designs will help optimize engineered bone regeneration.

6 Biologically-Based Scaffolds

Of the many different materials that could be used for biological bone scaffolds, hydroxyapatite (HA) is considered the most promising since it is a very strong osteoinductive factor [4]. The chemical formula for hydroxyapatite is $Ca_{10}(PO_4)_6(OH)_2$. Other materials containing calcium phosphate have been used as biomaterials for bone repair and regeneration [4]. The main advantage of using materials like hydroxyapatite, or any other synthetic calcium phosphate biomaterial is that these materials are much more biocompatible and stable than other synthetic materials when implanted in the body [4].

Although calcium phosphate biomaterials are better at regenerating bone, and are therefore promising bone substitute materials, these materials are inherently brittle in nature. This problem is generally solved by combining the crystalline biomaterials with polyesters [4]. This produces a scaffold that has the strong osteoinductive nature of the calcium phosphates, combined with the biodegradable and reactive nature of polyesters, allowing cell attachment to occur. To this end, many investigations with calcium phosphates or hydroxyapatite in combination with poly(ε-caprolactone) (PLC) or poly(lactide) (PLA) have been performed to produce potential bone substitutes [4]. It is hypothesized that the osteoinductive effects of these scaffolds can be attributed to their structural similarity to the extracellular matrix content of endogenous bone.

The mechanical properties of biologically-based bone scaffolds can also be modulated by cross-linking with different compounds [4]. For instance, it has been shown that crosslinking of calcium sulfate and poly(propylene fumarate) produces a scaffold with mechanical properties close to that of cortical bone, with a compressive strength of 5 MPa [4, 42]. In a different study, cross-linking with atelocollagen produced an injectable form of a bone substitute, which could be more effective for clinical use than implantable scaffolds. Hydroxyapatite-atelocollagen cross-linked compounds have been shown to promote ossification [4, 43]. However, despite this

Table 2 Mechanical properties of biologically-based scaffolds [39]

Polymer	Tensile strength (MPa)	Modulus (GPa)
HA/poly-caprolactone	20–43	0.4
poly(propylene fumarate)	2–30	2–3

compound's beneficial effects on bone regeneration, it's injectable nature makes it degrade rapidly and thus inadequate mechanically *in-vivo* [4]. As well, it was observed that hydroxyapatite particles in scaffolds tend to migrate to the surface and form clusters, which disturbs the homogeneity of the scaffold created initially [4]. A summary of the mechanical properties of the scaffolds described above is shown in Table 2.

6.1 Micro-Scale Properties of Scaffolds

In addition to cross-linking, the introduction of growth factors to a scaffold has been investigated. Bone morphogenetic protein (BMP) and transforming growth factor (TGF) are considered important for regulating bone remodeling [4]. The use of these growth factors in scaffolds to promote osteogenesis depends highly on the micro-scale properties of the scaffold, including the chemical binding and interactions of the growth factors with cells and compounds making up the structure of the scaffold.

To choose the appropriate chemical compounds for a scaffold, the micro-scale properties of the scaffold must be taken into consideration. These properties will affect the adhesion potential within the scaffold, as well as cell proliferation, survival, and function. Therefore, scaffolds with micro-scale structures containing pores that allow cell growth and distribution are vital [4]. In addition to allowing cell maintenance, the pores within a scaffold should also allow for angiogenesis, especially when considering bone regeneration. Mechanically, the optimal compressive modulus for hard and soft scaffolds range from 10–1500 MPa, and 0.4–350 MPa, respectively [44]. The complex relationship between scaffold porosity, rate of degradation, overall mechanical strength, and matching the scaffold surface to the properties of the surrounding bone still needs to be investigated before an engineered scaffold can be created that meets the mechanical demands of *in-vivo* bone.

6.2 Conclusions

From the evidence presented above, it seems that the production of an optimal biologically-based scaffold would encompass a structure that provides initial mechanical stability, stimulates ossification, and then gradually degrades as healing takes place. Choosing an appropriate material is fundamental to this process. Since scaffolds composed of mainly calcium phosphates are brittle, a material that is based on a polyester or gel modified with different compositions of calcium phosphate crystals would likely produce a three-dimensional, controlled structure capable of enhancing bone regeneration.

In order to produce a scaffold that also fulfills its biological demands, introducing mesenchymal or embryonic stem cells into tested scaffolds has been proposed. The foundation of this strategy would be to provide the bone defect with cells capable of either repairing the injured bone, or enhancing the ability of surrounding cells to remodel the defect in response to local mechanical signals.

7 Stem Cell Mechanobiology

The two main characteristics of stem cells are their ability to self potentiate, and their ability to differentiate. These characteristics are governed by what is called a "stem cell niche," a microenvironment in tissue where stem cells reside indefinitely while dividing into progenitor cells [45–47]. It is thought that cells no longer in self-renewal undergo differentiation, guided by factors within this "stem cell niche" that dictate their fate [45, 47, 48]. The different factors and signaling molecules involved in lineage determination has been extensively studied, but the role of mechanical factors in guiding stem cell fate is still unknown [47, 48]. Three mechanisms are believed to be involved in stem cell response to mechanical stress: direct cell-generated forces due to changes in the cytoskeleton, cell response due to the change in stiffness of the surrounding environment, and response due to the effect of external mechanical forces, such as gravity or muscle contraction [45–48].

The study of mechanobiology is essential to load-bearing tissues, such as the skeleton [47]. Stem cell-based regenerative strategies that aim to incorporate mechanical stimulation offer a controllable mechanical environment where the optimal environment for promoting stem cell differentiation can be determined [47, 48]. In terms of the musculoskeletal system, mesenchymal stem cells (MSCs) have been the most extensively studied [47]. It has been speculated that undifferentiated MSCs, which are responsible for development into bone, are responsive to mechanical stimulation mediated through the extracellular matrix [46–48]. For instance, it has been shown that increasing collagen concentration in the matrix surrounding cells results in MSC differentiation into an osteogenic lineage [47, 49].

Despite the promising research in MSCs, the ability of embryonic stem (ES) cells to divide indefinitely and differentiate into multiple tissue types make them equally attractive alternatives in modern tissue engineering [46, 47, 49]. Recent studies have shown that mechanical strain inhibits the differentiation of human ES cells while promoting self-renewal, as well as induces the production and diffusion of calcium and nitric oxide [47, 48]. Interestingly, these stem cells, cultured while being cyclically strained, retained pluripotency [47, 48]. This response to mechanical loading was hypothesized to involve the TGF-β signaling pathway, as the mechanical stimulus resulted in upregulation of TGF-β [48]. Thus, the influence of mechanical loading on stem cell response appears to depend on the type of stem cell as well as the state of differentiation. To this effect, it has been shown that the state of differentiation of human osteoblasts affected their responses to stretch loading *in vitro* [50]. Two effects of stretch were observed: induction of apoptosis, and induction of proliferation. The proliferative response to stretch was only observed in osteoblasts in a late maturation phase, from day 14 onwards [50]. The apoptotic response to stretch was observed in osteoblasts in an early phase of maturation [50]. The combined influence of differentiation and mechanical loading in regulating apoptosis and proliferation of bone cells seems to be an important mechanism involved in adaptation and remodeling in bone [48, 50]. In the same study where the effects of stretch (apoptotic and proliferative) were induced, the authors also showed that osteoblasts exhibiting high levels of alkaline phosphatase activity responded to mechanical loading by increasing cell numbers [50]. In addition, the apoptosis induced in early differentiated cultures and the protective effect in older cultures showed that the response of bone cells was independent of the osteogenic factors in the medium [50]. In these experiments, strain levels that induced osteoblast proliferation ranged from 0.1 % to 1 %, while strain levels higher than 5 % induced cell apoptosis [50]. In addition to endogenous matrix formation, the cells used in these experiments were also supplemented with collagen-I to facilitate adherence of the cells [50]. Because of this, it was hypothesized that during differentiation, as cells produced an extracellular matrix, some degree of shielding from the mechanical loading occurred. Although this shielding effect would not have affected the individual cell responses, the authors believed that it would affect the results of mechanical loading observed at the different stages of differentiation [50]. For instance, a certain level of differentiation was required to cause a proliferative response to stretch in the osteoblasts. Thus, the authors hypothesized that the sensitivity of the osteoblasts to mechanical loading changed during differentiation and may have reflected a difference in expression of a mechanosensing molecule in the extracellular matrix [50].

Therefore, regulation of apoptosis and proliferation by the combined influences of differentiation and mechanical forces can be an important mechanism involved in bone response and adaptation to mechanical loading. Given these findings, further investigation into the role of osteoblast differentiation as a regulator of a mechanotransduction molecule in bone, as well as the mediation of mechanical responses at different stages of differentiation is necessary to understand the complex signals and biochemical responses in bone adaptation and remodeling.

8 Models for Bone Repair

The need for greater mechanobiological understanding of stem cells and bone healing for tissue engineering therapies is essential to meet the clinical demand for novel strategies targeted towards the healing of acute bone defects [51, 52]. Even in healthy bone, the process of healing is complex both mechanically and biologically, with coordination required from multiple cell types including stem cells, osteoblasts, osteoclasts, and osteocytes [51]. Therefore, both traditional *in-vitro* approaches involving controlled mechanical stimulation, as well as *in-vivo* regenerative clinical approaches are necessary to understand and augment mechanically sensitive healing processes in bone [51].

8.1 In-vitro Models

For the study of highly specific research questions about the healing process of bone, *in-vitro* models are very relevant [51, 53, 54]. Most of the progress in these experiments stem from examining the mechanical sensitivity of bone healing in 2D cell culture systems [51, 53]. Many studies involving mesenchymal stem cells have shown that biaxial strain promoted osteogenic differentiation [51, 53]. Larger strains seemed to cause differentiated cells to de-differentiate and proliferate, while guiding undifferentiated cells to an osteogenic state [51, 53, 54].

Fluid shear stress has also been applied in 2D cell culture systems [51, 53, 54]. Most of these experiments used parallel plate chambers to apply the mechanical stimulus [51, 53]. In osteoblasts and osteocytes, it is believed that primary cilia on these cells are involved in mechanosensing fluid shear stress [51, 53]. The microtubule network in osteoblasts is also thought to be involved, where substrate deformation due to mechanical stress and fluid flow are thought to be linked to the response of osteoblasts in the healing process of bone [51, 53, 54]. Other *in-vitro* studies in 2D cell culture systems using cell poking, twisting, or pipette aspiration as the form of mechanical stimulation have provided valuable insight into the mechanical behavior of bone cells, but given the form of the mechanical stimulation, are harder to relate directly to the mechanical environment experienced by bone cells *in-vivo* [51, 53, 54].

In studies of bone regeneration, there continues to be a lack of emphasis on investigations of the specific character and magnitude of mechanical stimulation experienced in bone at a cellular level, as well as combining this knowledge with investigations of the biological factors involved in mechanosensing [51]. It is therefore generally agreed upon that in order to understand and develop tissue-level solutions for bone defects and pathologies, the cell culture environment is inadequate, and the need to transition to a 3-dimensional approach is necessary [51, 53, 54].

Culturing cells in 3D scaffolds can help model a physiological process [51, 54]. *In-vitro* models of the long bone healing environment have been modeled using mesenchymal stem cells seeded in a fibrin scaffold to represent a blood clot [51]. These studies subjected these cell-scaffold systems to a cyclic compressive load [51]. Results from the loading regime showed increased presence of collagen IX, a marker for calcification and endochondral ossification in bone [51]. In 3D cell scaffolds, the property of the substrate used for the scaffold has been shown to modify and determine stem cell lineage [51, 54]. Stiffer substrates have been shown to promote osteogenic differentiation of stem cells in a scaffold, whether they be mesenchymal or embryonic [51, 53, 54]. *In-vitro*, mechanically loaded constructs show greater levels of mineralization when the substrates for the scaffold have increased collagen and calcium content which contributes to overall construct stiffness [51]. In fact, under mechanical stimulation, it was found that nodules of mineralization could be found in very localized areas of strain [51]. Fluid flow applied *in-vitro* on cells within 3D scaffolds has also been shown to enhance mineralization and differentiation of stem cells into bone cells, due to the effects of both mechanical loading and improved transport of metabolites in a well structured three dimensional environment [51, 53, 54]. Using this knowledge, *in-vitro* culture models of *ex-vivo* tissue may offer additional insight and inspiration for novel approaches to bone regenerative medicine [51].

8.2 *In-vivo Models*

Several *in-vivo* stem cell studies have shown the benefit of applying implanted stem cells to the repair of a tissue [55–57]. Zhang et al. showed that bone marrow stem cells, when combined *in-vitro* with a fibrin extracellular glue, were capable of forming new bone in areas of alveolar bone defects in rats [55]. Healing was measurable as early as six weeks following *in-vivo* implantation, and the quantity of new bone formed was significantly greater than untreated and control groups [55]. Similarly, experiments by Kim et al. showed that xenogenic bone marrow stem cells were capable of surviving and contributing to bone repair in rabbits where defects in the lumbar spine existed [56]. The stem cells used in this study were combined with a compression resistant synthetic scaffold before implantation. Using Y-chromosome staining (used to monitor the viability of the male rabbit-derived cells), viability of the implanted cells was demonstrated between 1 to 6 months following implantation [56]. Additionally, the synthetic matrix created for implantation was eventually resorbed in the defect, and the production of new, mature bone containing both osteoblasts and osteocytes was demonstrated histologically [56]. Finally, a study by Minamide et al. successfully showed that bone marrow stem cells cultured *in-vitro* and seeded in a collagen-I gel with hydroxyapatite was capable of producing new bone formation in rabbits containing spinal bone defects [57]. Histology further showed the implanted cell-gel fragments successfully integrated themselves with the native mature bone surrounding it [57]. However, some concentrations of cells with hydroxyapatite produced fibrous tissue [57]. In all of these studies, only macroscopic techniques to study the extent of repair were performed.

In addition to stem cell implantation *in-vivo*, studies have also been performed to investigate the influence of mechanical stimulation on the natural course of bone healing [51, 58–60, 62, 63]. Through these investigations, several important factors in bone healing outcome have been identified. The first challenge in controlling and augmenting bone healing is the amount of mechanical stability in the fracture site [52]. In fact, the amount of external callus formed is related to the amount of movement present at the fracture site [52]. In bone healing, fracture callous formation usually occurs due to flexibility remaining around the affected site [52, 59, 60]. The more flexible the fixation, the larger the callus that is formed [52, 59, 60]. However, having a larger callus in a bone defect does not translate to higher mechanical strength and stiffness once the tissue is healed, or increase the rate of healing [52, 59, 60]. Therefore, studies to determine the optimal stability to promote rapid and mechanically stable bone healing still need to be performed. Another challenge in optimizing bone healing is controlling the amount of movement within the fracture site [52, 59, 60]. Studies by Goodship and Kenwright showed that induced micro-movements on tibial fractures in sheep resulted in increased callus formation and stiffness compared to rigid fixation of the fracture [52, 59, 60]. The studies also showed that smaller induced micro-movements resulted in improvements in the mineralization and rate of repair of the fracture [52, 59, 60]. A third factor shown to affect the control of mechanically-induced bone formation from *in-vivo* studies is the strain rate and timing of mechanical loading [52, 59]. Goodship et al. were able to demonstrate that high strain rates promoted bone healing, especially when stimulation was provided in the proliferative phase of bone healing [52, 59]. In addition to the strain rate and timing, the number of loading cycles was found to affect the regeneration of bone [52, 59]. A high number of loading cycles was able to positively stimulate bone formation [52, 59]. Specifically, a 0.4 mm axial movement was found to be optimal for resulting in a callus with high bone mineral density and resistance to bending [52, 59].

A series of *in-vivo* studies by Rubin et al. have also demonstrated the anabolic effect of low magnitude, high frequency vibrational loading on bone [61]. Frequencies ranging from 15–90 Hz were shown to increase the anabolic response of bone as frequency was increased [61]. Specifically, the number of trabeculae, bone volume, trabecular thickness, bone stiffness, and strength all increased after this loading was applied. Interestingly, in mice, this loading also produced a reduction of adipogenesis by altering commitment of mesenchymal stem cells to adipocytes, providing a loading regime highly favoring osteogenesis [61].

The size of the fracture defect has also been shown to influence healing outcome in bone [52, 62, 63]. The larger the size of the defect, the greater the reduction in the bending stiffness of the healed bone [52, 62, 63]. For small gaps, larger induced micro-movements and strains stimulated larger callus formation [52, 62, 63]. As well, the type of loading used caused differences in the amount of bone healing observed [52]. Moderate compressive axial mechanical stimulation was found to promote bone healing, while shear force was found to result in delayed healing and sometimes nonunion at the fracture site [52, 62, 63]. Similar results were found in an osteotomy model of sheep tibia, where shear stress was found to delay healing compared to axial stimulation [52, 62]. Additionally, cyclic compression resulted in significantly more callus formation than tension loading [52, 62, 63]. Overall, *in-vivo* studies have examined the influence of mechanical stimulation on the end healing outcome in bone [52, 59, 60, 62, 63] and investigated the factors that play a role in optimizing mechanically-induced bone formation. However, for modern tissue engineering strategies, a better understanding of bone healing is necessary, and the role of mechanical stimulation in this process. In order to achieve this, the time course of bone healing needs to be examined more thoroughly, since each step of the healing process (inflammation, hematoma formation, callus formation, remodeling) is affected differently by mechanical stimulation [52, 62, 63]. Using well developed techniques such as histology, immunohistochemistry, multi-photon microscopy, and µCT in small animal models will enable investigation of the role of mechanical stimulation on individual and time-dependent healing processes in bone defects, as well as reduce the inter-animal variability plaguing large animal models [52, 62, 63].

9 Implanting Cells Within a Scaffold

Uniform seeding of cells within a scaffold is difficult to control, but is a fundamental step in generating functional tissues [64]. Various techniques are used to distribute cells uniformly throughout a scaffold. One technique called "static seeding" involves pipetting a cell suspension into a gel-like, or porous scaffold [64]. A second method called "perfusion seeding" has also been proposed. Careful attention to the seeding method is of paramount importance since stirring or introducing a high amount of shear stress on the cells can cause cell death before integration into the scaffold can occur. Being able to provide an efficient yet reproducible seeding technique is equally important to the composition and structure of the scaffold created. The end of this chapter will address a technique used by our research group to incorporate murine embryonic stem cells into a collagen-I scaffold, and our initial findings on the levels of cell communication in the presence and absence of mechanical stimulation as these cells are stimulated to form osteoblasts.

The basis for integrating embryonic stem cells with a collagen gel is to determine the physical factors driving stem cells to differentiate in a fracture callous. It is well established that there is an interconnected relationship between connexin-containing gap junctions, cadherins, and integrins in cell communication and the response of cells to mechanical stimulation. Thus, our focus is to determine the role of connexin-containing gap junctions, cadherins, and mechanical stimulation on the biosynthetic activity of embryonic stem cells stimulated to form osteoblasts in a three-dimensional collagen-I scaffold (a "cell-gel construct"), and on cells in an *ex-vivo* bone model.

The first step to characterizing our scaffold was to determine the overall gap junction activity present and compare these results to reported *in-vitro* osteoblasts during differentiation. To date, the activity of gap junctions in our cell-gel constructs at 5, 15, 20 and 30 days of differentiation has been determined through fluorescence recovery after photobleaching (FRAP), and the presence of osteoblast-cadherin, Cx-32, and Cx-43 has been determined at these time points using immunofluorescence (IF). FRAP is a method that measures the two dimensional diffusion of fluorescently labeled macromolecules in the cytoplasm, cell membrane, and organelles. Cells are incubated with a molecule that diffuses into the cell. Living cells possess an enzyme capable of cleaving part of the molecule, rendering it both fluorescent and impermeable so it cannot then leave the cell. These fluorescent molecules in a small region

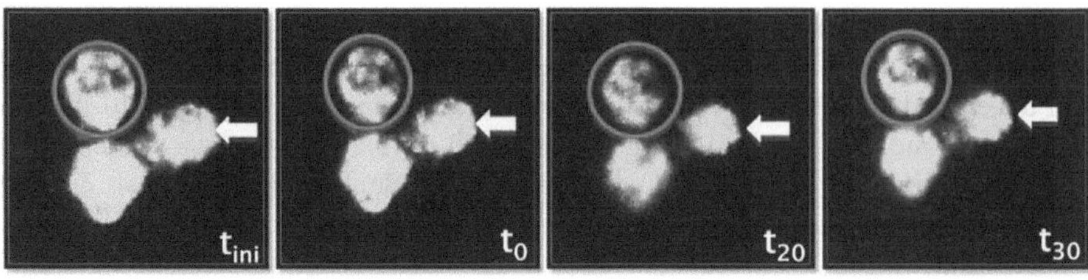

Fig. 1 Visualization of fluorescence recovery in cell-gel constructs before photobleaching (t_{ini}), after photobleaching (t_0), 20 minutes after photobleaching (t_{20}), and 30 minutes after photobleaching (t_{30}). *Red circle* indicates photobleached cell, *white arrow* indicates reference cell

of cells are irreversibly photobleached, causing a concentration gradient to form. If the bleached cell communicates with adjacent cells by means of gap junctions, this concentration gradient will be equilibrated. This equilibration is detected by monitoring fluorescence recovery (Fig. 1). It has been shown that calcein-AM is a good molecule for discriminating fluorescence recovery in short duration experiments. IF is a technique that enables the visualization of a specific protein or antigen in cells by binding a specific antibody that is fluorescently labeled.

9.1 Methods

Murine embryonic stem cells were maintained in T75 culture flasks, and after 3 to 4 passages, 1 million cells were spun down and resuspended in media containing pro-osteoblastic beta-glycerol phosphate (BGP) (260 mg/ml of media). The cells were then combined with purified bovine collagen I (Advanced BioMatrix, 800 µl collagen/1 ml cell-gel construct), seeded in 24-well plates, and incubated at 37 °C for 5, 15, 20, and 30 days. This protocol has been previously shown by our group to be sufficient for embryonic stem cell differentiation into osteoblasts in collagen gel constructs [65].

After 5, 15, 20, and 30 days of differentiation, cell-gel constructs were incubated at 37 °C with 500 µM calcein AM, or 1 mM octanol (a non-specific blocker of intercellular communication) for two hours. Constructs were also incubated in 100 µM α-glycyrrhetinic acid (a specific gap junction inhibitor) for 45 minutes to determine what effect specific gap junction blocking had on the ability of cells to communicate. A Zeiss LSM510 microscope was used for imaging. An initial image was recorded (t_{ini}) at 20 % laser intensity. An oval region of interest (ROI) was then fit around the cell body and any visible processes of a cell. This ROI was then photobleached at 100 % laser intensity for 10 to 15 seconds. Images were obtained immediately after photobleaching (t_0), after 2 min (t_2), 5 min (t_5), 10 min (t_{10}), 20 min (t_{20}), and 30 min (t_{30}) of recovery. The mean pixel intensity within cells was determined using NIH ImageJ 1.43 software and normalized to an uninvolved cell in the image field. Percent recovery for each image obtained after photobleaching was calculated using Eq. (1).

$$\%Recovery = \frac{(t_i - t_0)}{t_{ini}} \times 100 \tag{1}$$

After 5, 15, 20, and 30 days of differentiation, cell-gel constructs were also transferred to larger plates for immunofluorescence study. Each gel was fixed in filtered 4 % paraformaldehyde/PBS overnight at 4 °C. The gels were then washed three times in 1xPBS and incubated with filtered 0.5 % saponin/PBS overnight at 4 °C. The gels were washed again three times in 1xPBS and blocked overnight at 4 °C with 3 % BSA/PBS. After the blocking step, one gel was incubated with goat osteoblast-cadherin primary antibody, while two were incubated with mouse connexin-32 and connexin-43 primary antibody at a dilution of 1:50 in 3 % BSA/PBS overnight at 4 °C. The gels were then washed three times in 1xPBS and blocked again overnight at 4 °C in 3 % BSA/PBS. The gel with OB-Cad primary antibody was then incubated with anti-goat Alexa488 secondary antibody, and the gels with connexin primary antibodies were incubated in anti-mouse Alexa488 secondary antibody at a dilution of 1:50 in 3 % BSA/PBS. Finally, each gel was washed three times in 1xPBS and visualized using a Zeiss LSM510 microscope. One set of gels was not incubated in primary antibody to serve as a negative control. A pre-osteoblast cell line previously shown to have osteoblast-cadherin, connexin-32, and connexin-43 was used as a positive control. Fluorescence intensity of the cells at 10× magnification was measured using NIH ImageJ 1.43 software.

Additionally, confined compression of the cell-gel constructs was performed at the same time points using a custom designed FlexCell loading device with a loading regime of 4 hours per day for two days at a strain rate of 1 %, and a frequency of 1 Hz (Fig. 2). FRAP with and without AGA treatment was then performed on the loaded constructs to compare any differences in gap junction activity subsequent to mechanical loading.

9.2 Results

At an early stage (day 5), fluorescence recovery was approximately 8.42 %, whereas at each later stage of differentiation, recovery increased approximately two-fold. Octanol treatment resulted in an average percent recovery of 2.56 % ($n = 8$), while AGA treatment resulted in a 4.82 % recovery ($n = 12$). These values are likely attributable to movement of calcein labeled molecules within the photobleached cell, rather than additional fluorescent molecules diffusing to the photobleached cell from an adjacent cell. Using an independent two-sample t-test (assuming unequal sample size, and unequal sample variance), differences between average maximum percent recovery in early and late-differentiated murine osteoblasts is significant at $\alpha = 0.05$ ($p = 0.006$). This indicates that there is a significant difference in the activity of gap junctions in murine osteoblasts, with early differentiated osteoblasts exhibiting a lower gap junction activity than late differentiated osteoblasts.

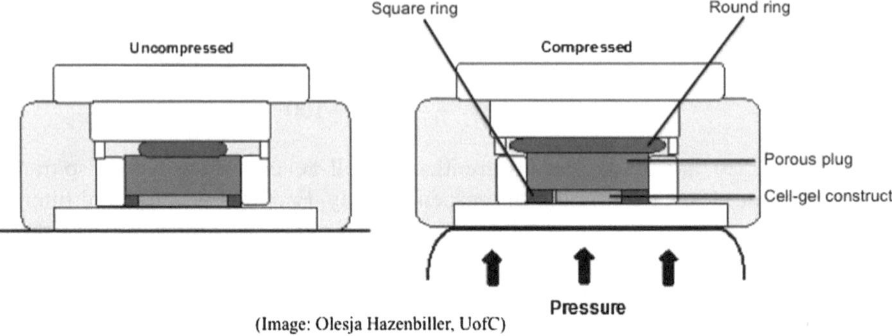

Fig. 2 FlexCell device for confined compression of cell-gel constructs

Immunofluorescence results showed greater presence of osteoblast-cadherin, connexin-32, and connexin-43 in day 15, day 20, and day 30 differentiated murine osteoblasts compared to day 5 differentiated murine osteoblasts. Images of the negative control did not show any presence of osteoblast-cadherin, connexin-32 and connexin-43, while images of the positive control demonstrated that the protocol was sufficient in revealing osteoblast-cadherin, connexin-32 and connexin-43 presence in the cell-gel constructs.

When mechanical stimulation was added, overall fluorescence recovery significantly increased by two-fold in day 5 constructs, but not in day 15, day 20, or day 30 constructs. FRAP of cell-gel constructs with AGA resulted in a lowered fluorescence recovery indicating successful inhibition of communication, and mechanical stimulation had no significant effect on this inhibition. When fluorescence recovery values in cell-gel constructs without AGA were investigated further, it was found that at 2 minutes after photobleaching, day 5 and day 20 constructs recovered significantly more fluorescence than the other stages of differentiation. The findings from these experiments are preliminary and will be investigated further.

9.3 Significance of This Tissue-Engineering Strategy for Bone

The developed preparation of embryonic stem cells within a collagen-I scaffold demonstrates a protocol that is reproducible, enables the formation of intercellular bonds and communication, and is responsive to mechanical stimulation. This novel strategy presents a scaffold preparation that is useful for further investigation of bone mechanobiology since the loading regime proposed can be controlled to alter the strain applied to the cell-gel construct. Any subsequent changes in fluid flow through the gel, as well as changes in cell behavior can then be investigated in this 3-dimensional construct. Transplanting this soft, porous, and hydrated scaffold into an *ex-vivo* bone defect model, and modulating the activity of gap junctions and cadherins will provide further insight into the role of cell communication on bone repair. Addition of mechanical stimulation to the *ex-vivo* construct with and without the implant will also lend insight into the role of mechanical stimulation on the repair of an acute bone defect.

10 Conclusion

The research reviewed here on stem cell-based approaches to tissue engineering of bone, together with the strategy proposed for incorporating osteoblastic cells into a collagen-I environment, illustrates advancing research that will provide an understanding of the importance of cell communication and the role of mechanical stimulation in the healing process of bone tissue. The biological and mechanistic insights derived from these studies may then be applied to developing strategies for stem cell-based healing of other acute injuries and chronic diseases.

The present work benefited from the input of Dr. John R. Matyas, Dr. Derrick E. Rancourt, and Dr. Roman Krawetz, who provided protocols and antibodies suitable for our study, and valuable criticism of the research summarized here. This research is supported by the Canadian Institute of Health Research, Alberta Innovates Technology Futures (GSS), and a Canada Research Chair in Orthopaedic Bioengineering (N.A.D.).

References

1. Marks SC, Popoff SN (1988) Bone cell biology: the regulation of development, structure, and function in the skeleton. Am J Anat 183:1–44
2. Willie BM, Petersen A, Schmidt-Bleek K et al (2010) Designing biomimetic scaffolds for bone regeneration: why aim for a copy of mature tissue properties if nature uses a different approach? Soft Matter 6:4976–4987
3. McKibbin B (1978) The biology of fracture healing in long bones. J Bone Jt Surg 60-B(2):150–162
4. Arvidson K, Abdallah BM, Applegate LA et al (2011) Bone regeneration and stem cells. J Cell Mol Med 15(4):718–746
5. Marsh D (1998) Concepts of fracture union, delayed union, and nonunion. Clin Orthop Relat Res 355:S22–S30
6. Anglen J (2002) Enhancement of fracture healing with bone stimulators. Tech Orthop 17(4):506–514
7. D'Aubigne RM (1949) Surgical treatment of nonunion of long bones. J Bone Jt Surg 31:256–266
8. AAOS (2007) Nonunions. American Academy of Orthopedic Surgeons, Rosemont. http://orthoinfo.aaos.org/topic.cfm?topic=A00374. Cited 15 Feb 2012
9. Crockett JC, Rogers MJ, Coxon FP et al (2011) Bone remodelling at a glance. J Cell Sci 124:991–998

10. Batra N, Kar R, Jiang J (2011) Gap junctions and hemichannels in signal transmission, function and development of bone. Biochim Biophys Acta. doi:10.1016/j.bbamem.2011.09.018

11. Jiang JX, Siller-Jackson AJ, Burra S (2007) Roles of gap junctions and hemichannels in bone cell functions and in signal transmission of mechanical stress. Front Biosci 12:1450–1462

12. Stains JP, Civitelli R (2005) Gap junctions in skeletal development and function. Biochim Biophys Acta 1719:69–81

13. Ishihara Y, Kamioka H, Honjo T et al (2008) Hormonal, pH, and calcium regulation of connexin 43-mediated dye transfer in osteocytes in chick calvaria. J Bone Miner Res 23(3):350–360

14. Matemba SF, Lie A, Ransjo M (2006) Regulation of osteoclastogenesis by gap junction communication. J Cell Biochem 99(2):528–537

15. Watkins M, Grimston SK, Norris JY et al (2011) Osteoblast connexin 43 modulates skeletal architecture by regulating both arms of bone remodelling. Mol Biol Cell 22:1240–1251

16. Su M, Borke JL, Donahue HJ et al (1997) Expression of connexin 43 in rat mandibular bone and periodontal ligament cells during experimental tooth movement. J Dent Res 76:1357–1366

17. Cheng B, Zhao S, Luo J et al (2001) Expression of functional gap junctions and regulation by fluid flow shear stress in osteocyte-like MLO-Y4 cells. J Bone Miner Res 16:249–259

18. Civitelli R (2008) Cell-cell communication in the osteoblast/osteocyte lineage. Biochem Biophys 473:188–192

19. Genetos DC, Geist DJ, Liu D et al (2005) Fluid shear-induced ATP secretion mediates prostaglandin release in MC3T3-E1 osteoblasts. J Bone Miner Res 20:41–49

20. Dale B, Gualtieri R, Talevi R et al (1991) Intercellular communication in the early human embryo. Mol Reprod Dev 29(1):21–28

21. Mbalaviele G, Shin CS, Civitelli R (2006) Cell-cell adhesion and signaling through cadherins: connecting bone cells in their microenvironment. J Bone Miner Res 21(12):1821–1827

22. Schwartz MA, DeSimone DW (2008) Cell adhesion receptors in mechanotransduction. Curr Opin Cell Biol 20:551–556

23. Pokutta S, Weis WI (2007) Structure and mechanism of cadherins and catenins in cell-cell contacts. Annu Rev Cell Dev Biol 23:237–261

24. Ganz A, Lambert M, Saez A et al (2006) Traction forces exerted through N-cadherin contacts. Biol Cell 98:721–730

25. Leucht P, Kim JB, Currey JA et al (2007) FAK-mediated mechanotransduction in skeletal regeneration. PLoS ONE 2:e390

26. Rhee ST, El-Bassiony L, Buchman SR (2006) Extracellular signal-related kinase and bone morphogenetic protein expression during distraction osteogenesis of the mandible: in vivo evidence of a mechanotransduction mechanism for differentiation and osteogenesis by mesenchymal precursor cells. Plast Reconstr Surg 117:2243–2249

27. Duong LT, Lakkakorpi P, Nakamura I et al (2000) Integrins and signaling in osteoclast function. Matrix Biology 19:97–105

28. Houghton FD (2005) Role of gap junctions during early embryo development. Reproduction 129(2):129–135

29. Nakamura I, Duong LT, Rodan SB et al (2007) Involvement of alpha-v-beta-3 integrins in osteoclast function. J Bone Miner Metab 25:337–344

30. Pioletti DP (2010) Biomechanics in bone tissue engineering. Comput Methods Biomech Biomed Eng 13(6):837–846

31. Juncosa N, West JR, Galloway MT et al (2003) In vivo forces used to develop design parameters for tissue engineered implants for rabbit patellar tendon repair. J Biomech 36:483–488

32. Tate ML, Knothe U (2000) An ex vivo model to study transport processes and fluid flow in loaded bone. J Biomech 33:247–254

33. Blecha LD, Rakotomanana L, Razafimahery F et al (2009) Targeted mechanical properties for optimal fluid motion inside artificial bone substitutes. J Orthop Res 27:1082–1089

34. Behravesh E, Yasko AW, Engel PS et al (1999) Synthetic biodegradable polymers for orthopaedic applications. Clin Orthop 367S:118–129

35. Stevens MM, Marini RP, Schaefer D et al (2005) In vivo engineering of organs: the bone bioreactor. Proc Natl Acad Sci USA 102:11450–11455
36. Li F, Li S, Ghzaoui AE et al (2007) Synthesis and gelation properties of PEG-PLA-PEG triblock copolymers obtained by coupling monohydroxylated PEG-PLA with adipoyl chloride. Langmuir 27:2778–2783
37. Ryner M, Albertsson AC (2002) Resorbable and highly elastic block copolymers from 1,5-dioxepan-2-one and L-lactide with controlled tensile properties and hydrophilicity. Biomacromolecules 3:601–608
38. Ryner M, Valdre A, Albertsson AC (2002) Star-shaped and photo-crosslinked poly(1,5-dioxepan-2-one)—synthesis and characterization. J Polym Sci, Part A, Polym Sci 40:2049–2054
39. Iqbal M, Xu X (2009) A review on biodegradable polymeric materials for bone tissue. J Mater Sci 44(51):5713–5724
40. Swaminathan V, Tchao R, Jonnalaggada S (2007) Physical characterization of thin semi-porous poly(L-lactic acid)/poly(ethylene glycol) membranes for tissue engineering. J Biomater Sci Polym Ed 18(10):1321–1333
41. Kroeze RJ, Helder MN, Govaert LE et al (2009) Biodegradable polymers in bone tissue engineering. Materials 2:833–856
42. Cai ZY, Yang DA, Zhang N et al (2009) Poly(propylene-fumarate)/(calcium sulfate/β-tricalcium phosphate) composites: preparation, characterization and in-vitro degradation. Acta Biomater 5:628–635
43. Pelin IM, Maier SS, Chitanu GC et al (2009) Preparation and characterization of a hydroxyapatite-collagen composite as component for injectable bone substitute. Mater Sci Eng 29:2188–2194
44. Hollister SJ (2005) Porous scaffold design for tissue engineering. Nat Mater 4:518–524
45. Alessandri G, Emanueli C, Madeddu P (2004) Genetically engineered stem cell therapy for tissue regeneration. Ann NY Acad Sci 1015:271–284
46. Rahaman MN, Mao JJ (2005) Stem cell-based composite tissue constructs for regenerative medicine. Biotechnol Bioeng 91:261–284
47. Lee DA, Knight MM, Campbell JJ et al (2011) Stem cell mechanobiology. J Cell Biochem 112:1–9
48. Guilak F, Cohen DM, Estes BT et al (2009) Control of stem cell fate by physical interactions with the extracellular matrix. Cell Stem Cell 5:17–26
49. Battista S, Guarnieri D, Borselli C et al (2005) The effect of matrix composition of 3D constructs on embryonic stem cell differentiation. Biomaterials 26:6194–6207.
50. Weyts FA, Bosmans B, Niesing R et al (2003) Mechanical control of human osteoblast apoptosis and proliferation in relation to differentiation. Calcif Tissue Int 4:505–512
51. Thompson MS, Epari DR, Bieler F et al (2010) In vitro models for bone mechanobiology: applications in bone regeneration and tissue engineering. Proc Inst Mech Eng 224:1533–1541
52. Epari DR, Duda GN, Thompson MS (2010) Mechanobiology of bone healing and regeneration: in vivo models. Proc Inst Mech Eng 224:1543–1553
53. Ziambaras K, Lecanda F, Steinberg TH et al (1998) Cyclic stretch enhances gap junctional communication between osteoblastic cells. J Bone Miner Res 13(2):218–228
54. Grimston SK, Screen J, Haskell JH et al (2006) Role of connexin 43 in osteoblast response to physical load. Ann NY Acad Sci 1068:214–224
55. Zhang L, Wang P, Mei S et al (2011) In vivo alveolar bone regeneration by bone marrow stem cells/fibrin glue composition. Oral Biology. doi:10.1016/j.archoralbio.2011.08.025
56. Kim H, Park J, Lee JK et al (2008) Transplanted xenogenic bone marrow stem cells survive and generate new bone formation in the posterolateral lumbar spine of non-immunosuppressed rabbits. Eur Spine J 17:1515–1521
57. Minamide A, Yoshida M, Kawakami M et al (2005) The use of cultured bone marrow cells in type I collagen gel and porous hydroxyapatite for posterolateral lumbar spine fusion. Spine 30(10):1134–1138

58. Grimston SK, Brodt MD, Silva MJ et al (2008) Attenuated response to in vivo mechanical loading in mice with conditional osteoblast ablation of the connexin 43 gene (GJA1). J Bone Miner Res 23(6):879–886
59. Goodship AE, Kenwright J (1985) The influence of induced micromovement upon the healing of experimental tibial fractures. J Bone Jt Surg 67(4):650–655
60. Kenwright J, Goodship AE (1989) Controlled mechanical stimulation in the treatment of tibial fractures. Clin Orthop Relat Res 241:36–47
61. Rubin C, Judex S, Qin YX (2006) Low-level mechanical signals and their potential as a non-pharmacological intervention for osteoporosis. Age Ageing 35(S2):32–36
62. Augat P, Merk J, Wolf S et al (2001) Mechanical stimulation by external application of cyclic tensile strains does not effectively enhance bone healing. J Orthop Trauma 15(1):54–60
63. Hente R, Fuchtmeier B, Schlegel U et al (2004) The influence of cyclic compression and distraction on the healing of experimental tibial fractures. J Orthop Res 22(4):709–715
64. Wang X, Nyman JS, Dong X et al (2010) Fundamental biomechanics in bone tissue engineering. doi:10.2200/S00246ED1V01Y200912TIS004
65. Krawetz R, Cormier J, Wu Y et al (2011) Collagen I scaffolds cross-linked with beta-glycerol phosphate induce osteogenic differentiation of embryonic stem cells in vitro and regulates their tumorigenic potential in vivo. Tissue Eng, Part A. doi:10.1089/ten.TEA.2011.0174

In Silico Biology of Bone Regeneration Inside Calcium Phosphate Scaffolds

Aurélie Carlier, Hans Van Oosterwyck, and Liesbet Geris

Abstract Bone tissue engineering plays a key role in finding better solutions for the healing of large bone defects and non-unions. Despite extensive experimental research, many of the mechanisms of the bone regeneration process still remain to be elucidated. As such, mathematical modeling is a useful tool to further investigate the different influential factors and their interactions *in silico*. This chapter starts with a description of the biological processes that take place during bone regeneration in calcium phosphate (CaP) scaffolds. The second section gives an overview of the most recent mathematical models of bone regeneration in (CaP) scaffolds. One model is explained in more detail and used to illustrate the potential of mathematical modeling in the bone tissue engineering field. Finally, the drawbacks of the current modeling techniques and the need for more quantitative experimental research, together with possible solutions are presented.

1 Introduction

The need for bone tissue regeneration is continuously increasing due to the improvement of the quality of life and the increase in life expectancy. In the United States alone approximately 6 million fractures occur yearly, of which 5–10 % result in a delayed union or in a non-union. An extrapolation of these numbers to the Indian population results in 240 million fractures a year, of which 12 million non-unions [4]. Bone tissue engineering aims at finding a better solution for the healing of large bone defects and non-unions. This interdisciplinary research field applies principles of engineering and life sciences to create an *in vivo* micro-environment that

A. Carlier (✉) · H. Van Oosterwyck
Biomechanics Section, KU Leuven, Celestijnenlaan 300C, PB 2419, 3001 Heverlee, Belgium
e-mail: aurelie.carlier@mech.kuleuven.be

H. Van Oosterwyck
e-mail: hans.vanoosterwyck@mech.kuleuven.be

L. Geris
Biomechanics Research Unit, U. Liège, Chemin de Chevreuils 1, PB 52/3, 4000 Liège, Belgium
e-mail: liesbet.geris@ulg.ac.be

P.R. Fernandes, P.J. Bártolo (eds.), *Tissue Engineering*,
Computational Methods in Applied Sciences 31, DOI 10.1007/978-94-007-7073-7_2,
© Springer Science+Business Media Dordrecht 2014

promotes local bone repair or regeneration [14, 19]. Bone formation is a very complex physiological process, involving the participation of many different cell types and regulated by countless biochemical and mechanical factors. Therefore, mathematical models can make a significant contribution in further unraveling the interactions between the different influential factors. Thus, *in silico* experimentation seeks to explain and understand the underlying principles of the biological phenomenon. Moreover, mathematical models can be used to design and test possible experimental and therapeutic strategies *in silico* before they are tested *in vitro* or *in vivo*. These experimental results will, in turn, guide further model building.

This book chapter will start with an overview of the biology of bone regeneration inside calcium phosphate (CaP) scaffolds. Then some mathematical models of bone regeneration inside (CaP) scaffolds will be discussed, indicating clearly the opportunities of an integrative approach that combines mathematical modeling with experimental research. Finally, some future prospects are presented.

2 Biology of Bone Regeneration Inside CaP Scaffolds

Tissue engineering aims to develop biological substitutes that restore, maintain or improve tissue function. Two main strategies have been developed to regenerate bone tissue: the use of biomaterials to induce bone formation chemically and the construction of hybrid implants composed of a biomaterial scaffold seeded with osteogenic cells [19, 25]. Delayed and non-unions are characterized by an *in vivo* micro-environment that fails to support bone repair or tissue regeneration. Hence, the micro-environment found at a non-union could be considered as an ectopic site [14]. Consequently, the tissue engineering constructs should display osteoinductive properties. CaP bioceramics are then interesting candidates, because of their biocompatibility, bioactivity and osteoinductive characteristics. It has been clearly shown that CaP induces bone formation, but the exact mechanism is still largely unknown [2, 10, 14, 20, 35, 46]. There are, however, several mechanisms proposed in literature to explain the influence of CaP particles on bone formation as observed in many experiments.

It has been stated that a high local concentration of growth factors and proteins can be achieved by adsorption on the biomaterial substrate, thereby creating a favorable micro-environment for bone formation [28, 35, 46]. Another explanation for the osteoinductive properties of CaP biomaterials is given by the surface topography, since it influences the osteoblastic guidance and attachment and can cause the asymmetrical division of MSCs [1, 2]. Barrère et al. [2] also suggest that the surface charge of the substrate can play a key role by triggering cell differentiation. Furthermore, negative charges distributed on the surface of the biomaterial can be an obstacle for cell-material adhesion, because the cell surface is also negatively charged [40, 47]. The bioapatite layer, formed *in vivo*, might also be recognized by MSCs [19]. A low oxygen tension in the central region of the biomaterial, which triggers the pericytes of microvessels to differentiate in osteoblasts, is another mechanism proposed in literature [2]. However, the release of calcium and phosphate ions by dissolution, is believed to be the main origin of the bioactivity of CaP biomaterials [1, 2, 10, 19]. The dissolution properties of CaP biomaterials are influenced by the exposed surface area, the composition and the pH. Pioletti et al. [34] showed that small CaP particles ($< 10 \, \mu m$) can induce phagocytosis. This process could then, in turn, produce an accumulation of Ca^{2+} in the mitochondria, which can cause lysis of the mitochondria and cell death. Phagocytosis also alters the pH of the surrounding body fluids. This pH-change subsequently alters the dissolution properties of the CaP particles. The size of the particles is not only critical because it can induce phagocytosis, it also determines the reactivity of the particles. The smaller the particles, the larger the exposed surface to the environment and the faster the biomaterial will dissolve. The dissolution rate will increase, simply because larger quantities of exchange can take place [1]. The composition of the calcium phosphate biomaterials is another important characteristic that determines the dissolution properties. A change in the calcium to phosphate ratio means a change in phase composition, which directly affects the ionic exchange mechanisms [1].

Experimental evidence clearly indicates the key role of calcium. Yuan et al. [53] observe more bone formation in scaffolds made up of biphasic CaP than of hydroxyapatite, the latter having a lower dissolution rate. The effect of calcium ion implantation in titanium on bone formation was investigated by Hanawa et al. [20]. They found a larger amount of new bone on the Ca^{2+}-treated side than on the untreated side. Eyckmans et al. [14] noticed that the CaP granule remnants in a decalcified scaffold serve as anchoring points for cell attachment. Titorencu et al. [44] report that osteoblasts respond to changes in Ca^{2+} concentration in the bone microenvironment. Moreover, differentiation of MSCs towards osteoblasts is accompanied by the expression of Ca^{2+} binding-proteins and the incorporation of Ca^{2+} into the extracellular matrix [44]. Chai et al. [9] observed a significant Ca^{2+}-induced cell proliferation and upregulation of osteogenic gene expression in a dose- and time-dependent manner. It also appears that osteoblasts sense and respond to the extracellular Ca^{2+} concentration independently of systemic calciotropic factors in a concentration-dependent manner [13]. Bootman et al. [7] report that the extracellular calcium concentration could control the frequency of the intracellular calcium spiking, which encodes specific cellular information according to Sun et al. [43].

The release of PO_4^{3-} also plays a key role by regulating the cell cycle and proliferation rate, influencing gene expression [3] and the secretion of bone-related proteins [23]. However, several *in vitro* studies showed that the addition of high levels of exogenous PO_4^{3-} (5–7 mM) induced osteoblast apoptosis and non-physiological mineral deposition [27]. Nevertheless, PO_4^{3-} is believed to play a critical role in bone matrix mineralization [32].

Despite of the vast *in vitro* research findings, the influences of Ca^{2+} and PO_4^{3-} differ from cell type to cell type. This implies that there will be not one optimal Ca^{2+} and P_i concentration that could universally drive all cell types towards successful osteogenesis. Moreover, the optimal concentration may vary according to the cellular stage, e.g. proliferation and differentiation. Therefore, specific windows of ion concentration need to be determined and optimized for a specific *in vitro* and *in vivo* response.

3 Mathematical Models of Bone Regeneration Inside (CaP) Scaffolds

3.1 From Models...

Improvements in computer capacity now enable an increased model realism and complexity (e.g. 3D calculations, complex geometries, multi-scale, multi-physics, ...) [45]. As a consequence of this technological revolution, there has been an enormous increase in the use of mathematical models in biology and medicine. These mathematical models can propose and test possible biological mechanisms, contributing to the unraveling of the complex nature of biological systems. Moreover, they can be used to design and test possible experimental strategies *in silico* before they are tested *in vitro* or *in vivo*. Finally, all this knowledge can be used to develop clinically relevant cell carriers.

Currently, many computational models of bone formation and regeneration in general (reviewed in Geris et al. [16–18]), or even in (CaP) scaffolds specifically (reviewed in Sengers et al. [39]) exist. Bohner et al. [6] propose a theoretical approach to determine the effect of geometrical factors on the resorption rate of CaP scaffolds. The theoretical model was based on five assumptions: (i) the pores are spherical, (ii) the pores follow a face-centered cubic packing, (iii) the resorption is surface-controlled, (iv) the resorption requires the presence of blood vessels (50 μm in diameter) and (v) the resorption time is proportional to the net amount of material [6]. Based on these assumptions the model calculations show that the resorption time of a macroporous block depends on the pore radius which is dependent on the size of the bone substitute and the interpore distance [6]. The model was also used to optimize the pore size of CaP scaffolds and validated with experimental data. The theoretical model looks, however, exclusively at geometrical scaffold properties and does not include biological variables such as cells or matrix densities. Byrne et al. [8] developed a 3D mechanoregulatory model of bone regeneration in a regular scaffold to investigate the effect of porosity, Young's modulus and dissolution rate on bone regeneration in different loading conditions. They model the scaffold degradation in a linear, load-independent fashion, i.e. the porosity will be increased by a 0 %, 0.5 %, 1 % per iteration for low, intermediate and high dissolution rates respectively [8]. Consequently, the size of all scaffold elements decreases uniformly resulting in an overall volumetric reduction while the scaffold geometry remains unaltered [8]. Their calculations show that as scaffold degradation progresses, the regenerating tissue must take over the mechanical function of the bone-scaffold system which would otherwise collapse due to a lack of mechanical strength [8]. Moreover, all three variables (i.e. porosity, Young's modulus and dissolution rate) appear to influence the amount of bone formation in a non-intuitive way, demonstrating the need to optimize scaffolds for site-specific loading requirements [8]. This model was improved by including blood vessel growth thereby establishing a framework to investigate the effect of vascularization on bone formation [12].

Other studies have modeled the bone regeneration process inside biodegradable polymer-based scaffolds. Stops et al. [42] further investigated the influence of mechanical strain and perfusive fluid flow on cell differentiation and proliferation within a collagen-glycosaminoglycan scaffold. Sanz-Herrera et al. [37] presented a multi-scale model of bone regeneration inside a porous scaffold. The biodegradable polymer scaffold degrades hydrolytically, i.e. the water content in the polymer chemically reacts and breaks down the material, which was modelled accordingly [37]. The mechanical properties of the polymer were assumed to relate linearly to its molecular weight [37]. The evolution of the bone formation process in a scaffold implanted in the femoral condyle of a rabbit was simulated with the model. They found a good qualitative agreement between the obtained computational and experimental results [37]. Although further validation is necessary, the proposed multi-scale model is a useful tool to investigate the complex phenomena that occur at different length and time scales, i.e. the bone formation and scaffold resorption at the microscopic scale and the change of mechanical properties at the macroscopic scale [37]. Lacroix et al. [24] nicely review the current techniques used for scaffold development: from scaffold optimization of scaffolds by mathematical models (e.g. FEM) to scaffold design using computer aided design (CAD) and scaffold characterization by computed tomography (CT).

Although the above models can be used to optimize some (mechanical) properties of scaffolds, e.g. the porosity, the micro-architecture, the Young's modulus and dissolution rate, they neglect the influence of growth factors and other biochemical signals on the bone formation process. Moreover, the dissolution process is only crudely modeled, neglecting the influence of the degradation products (e.g. Ca^{2+} and P_i) on the cellular activities and bone formation process. Carlier et al. [11] developed and implemented an experimentally informed bioregulatory model of the effect of calcium ions released from CaP-based biomaterials on the activity of osteogenic cells and mesenchymal stem cell driven ectopic bone formation. The model describes the effect of CaP biomaterials on the activity of osteogenic cells as a temporal variation of six variables: free extracellular Ca^{2+} concentration (Ca), MSC density (c_m), osteoblast density (c_b), mineral matrix density (b), collagen matrix density (m) and a generic, osteogenic growth factor concentration (g_b). The sum of the mineral matrix and the collagen matrix represents the total bone density. The evolution of each of these continuous variables is described by the following set of delay differential equations (DDEs) (see Fig. 1):

$$\frac{\partial c_m(t)}{\partial t} = \overbrace{A_m(t).c_m(t).\big(1 - \alpha_m.c_m(t)\big).\beta_{cm}(t)}^{proliferation} - \overbrace{F_1(t).c_m(t-t_1)}^{differentiation} - \overbrace{d(t)}^{removal}$$

$$\frac{\partial c_b(t)}{\partial t} = \overbrace{A_b(t).c_b(t).\big(1 - \alpha_b.c_b(t)\big).\beta_{cb}(t)}^{proliferation} + \overbrace{F_1(t).c_m(t-t_1)}^{differentiation} - \overbrace{d_b.c_b(t)}^{removal}$$

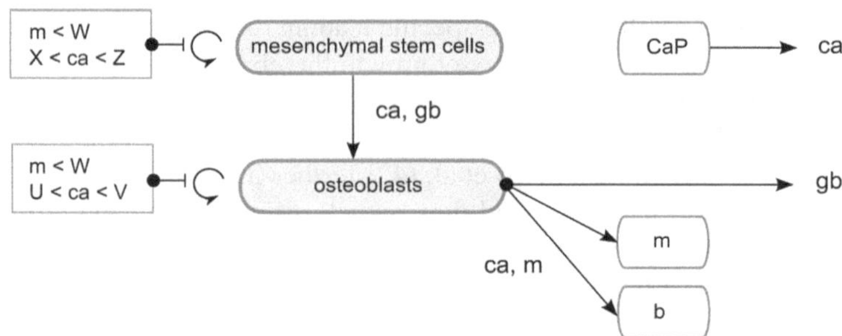

Fig. 1 Schematic overview of the calcium model. W = maximum tissue density for proliferation, X = minimum calcium concentration for proliferation of MSCs, Z = maximum calcium concentration for proliferation of MSCs, U = minimum calcium concentration for proliferation of osteoblasts, V = maximum calcium concentration for proliferation of osteoblasts, $ca = \mathrm{Ca}^{2+}$, gb = growth factor, m = osteoid, b = mineral matrix. The participation of a variable in a subprocess is indicated by showing the name of that variable next to the *arrow* representing that subprocess, e.g. calcium modulates differentiation and bone formation (adapted from Carlier et al. [11])

$$\frac{\partial m(t)}{\partial t} = \overbrace{P_{bs}.\big(1 - \kappa_b.m(t)\big).c_b(t - t_2)}^{\text{production}}$$

$$\frac{\partial b(t)}{\partial t} = \overbrace{P_{bb}.\big(1 - \delta - \kappa_{bb}.b(t)\big)^6.c_b(t)}^{\text{production}}$$

$$\frac{\partial g_b(t)}{\partial t} = \overbrace{E_{gb}(t).c_b(t)}^{\text{production}} - \overbrace{d_{gb}g_b(t)}^{\text{decay}} - \overbrace{R(t)}^{\text{consumption}}$$

$$\frac{\partial Ca(t)}{\partial t} = \overbrace{\sigma.\big(Ca_\infty - Ca(t)\big)}^{\text{release}} - \overbrace{J(t).c_b(t)}^{\text{consumption (HA)}} - \overbrace{d_{Ca}.Ca(t).\big(c_b(t) + c_m(t)\big)}^{\text{consumption (metabolism)}}$$

In short, cell differentiation is controlled by the presence of growth factors and calcium. The local cell and matrix densities, as well as the calcium concentration influence the proliferation of both MSCs and osteoblasts. Matrix synthesis is controlled by the local cell and matrix densities. The local cell and growth factor concentrations influence the growth factor production, whereas the calcium concentration depends on the dissolution rate of the CaP biomaterial and uptake by the osteogenic cells. The model equations are implemented in Matlab (The MathWorks, Inc.) using delay differential equations routines. Additional information, including an extensive discussion on the processes described by these equations, the boundary and initial conditions, parameter values and implementation details can be found in the Appendix (Tables 1 and 2) and in Carlier et al. [11].

Mathematical models have several advantages with respect to experimental research. The act of developing a model consists out of translating the biological processes into mathematical equations, which can be continuous, discrete or a hybrid variant. This process of translation is in itself very valuable since it requires a thorough understanding of the biological process under study. The modeler will need to decide which variables are most important to answer the research question at hand and how the underlying biological processes will be represented. Often this is done in close collaboration with experimental biologists who might have a different view and strategy of tackling problems. These very fundamental discussions and questions often lead to new insights and research tracks and are therefore a noteworthy advantage of mathematical modeling.

Mathematical models can also be used to compute information that would be impossible to obtain experimentally. For example, Milan et al. [31] use a finite element analysis to calculate the shear strain, fluid flow and pore pressures inside a porous polymeric scaffold. Also Byrne et al. [8] use a finite element analysis to compute the strain and fluid flow which are then used as input for the mechanoregulatory model of tissue differentiation. It is clear that these biophysical stimuli play a key role in the bone regeneration process. Besides the mechanoregulatory variables, also bioregulatory variables are difficult to measure in an *in vitro* or *in vivo* setting. Carlier et al. [11] calculate the amount of calcium that is released by the CaP scaffold and taken up by the osteogenic cells. Although this model is only one-dimensional, an extension with spatial dimensions would allow the determination of the calcium distribution inside the scaffold and developing tissue. This is important since calcium influences many cellular processes as was shown in the previous section.

The experimental difficulties mentioned above entail however problems for model validation. The results of a model have indeed no meaning if they are not corroborated by real *in vitro* or *in vivo* data. This problem is often solved by measuring related quantities and seeing how they correspond to the model predictions. Byrne et al. [8] suggest for example to implant a scaffold into a bone defect in an animal model and making histological measurements of tissue phenotype at several time points which could then be compared to the simulation results. Another technique is to use the model framework in a different application and determining whether the predictions also fit in this new setting. The model of Carlier et al. [11] was validated by comparison with experimental data. Firstly, it was found that the model of Carlier et al. [11] is able to reproduce the sequential events observed experimentally during intramembranous healing: (1) proliferation, (2) differentiation, (3) collagen production and (4) mineralization [29, 41]. Secondly, the model results were compared to the experimentally determined amount of bone formation by Hartman et al. [21]. It was found that the results of the simulation and the experiment correspond qualitatively. Thirdly, the modeling platform successfully predicted the absence of bone in the impaired healing situations of scaffold decalcification and insufficient cell seeding. However, the results of the model should be interpreted in a qualitative way due to some simplifications and parameter value estimations. The current tool would have much more potential if it could be made more quantitative. A major problem in that respect is the lack of extensive characterization and quantification of the scaffold properties. As such it is difficult to match the experimental conditions found in literature with the modeled ones. Currently, specific *in vivo* and *in vitro* testing procedures are being set up to determine the calcium release rate and relate it to the *in vivo* bone forming capacity of different CaP scaffolds.

                                                                A. Carlier et al.

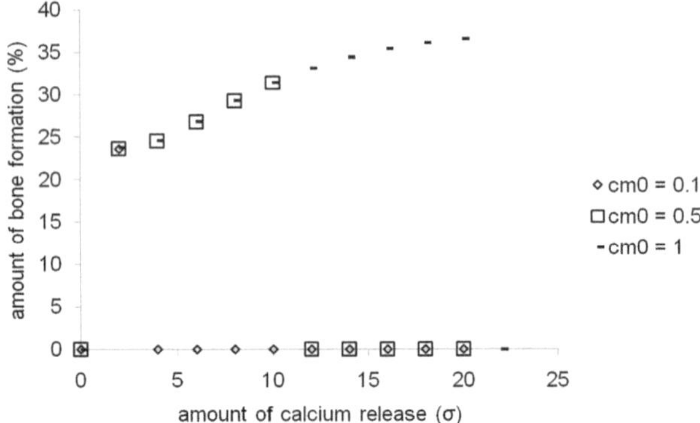

Fig. 2 Amount of bone formation at day 90 as a function of the calcium release rate (σ) and initial MSC concentration (c_{m0}) according to the mathematical model

After the development and validation of the model, the model needs to be further analyzed and can be used for optimization. The analysis phase allows determining which factors are the most important ones and how they interact. This is another major advantage of modeling. Since biological systems are so complex, it is often difficult to intuitively predict what will happen if a specific factor is changed. To determine the most influential factors of the mathematical model, Carlier et al. [11] performed a sensitivity analysis by "Design of Experiments" (DOE). DOE is a statistical tool that enables the determination of an efficient design for (in this case) a multi-parameter sensitivity analysis. Carlier et al. [11] used the JMP statistical software (8.0.1. SAS Institute Inc.) to generate the array of combinations of different parameter values within a pre-defined parameter space. The sensitivity analysis showed that the bone formation rate P_{bb}, the initial MSC density c_{m0} and the initial osteoblast density c_{b0} are the most important factors influencing the amount of bone formation at day 21 and 42 [11]. The model outcome also largely depends on the initial conditions, which therefore should be realistically defined. The sensitivity analysis indicated a significant interaction between the calcium release and the initial MSC seeding density which was subsequently further investigated (see Fig. 2). The model indicates that a low initial MSC density requires a low calcium release rate, while a high initial MSC density requires a high calcium release rate in order to maximize the amount of bone formation. The amount of bone formation for low initial MSC concentrations is also very sensitive to calcium, whereas high initial MSC concentrations produce similar amounts of bone for a range of calcium release. For tissue engineering strategies it is interesting to start with a low initial cell density but since the margin is very small, the optimization is critical for these types of constructs. The high MSC concentrations entail a larger window of allowable calcium release rates which allows for more optimization and potentially higher benefits. The *in vivo* bone formation capacity of different CaP scaffolds seeded with a fixed concentration of hPDCs was studied by Roberts et al. [36]. They found that the calcium release rate is a strong determinant in discriminating bone-forming scaffolds from scaffolds that did not lead to any bone formation thereby confirming our initial hypothesis. This integrative research shows that mathematical models can be used to determine whether a certain mechanism, proposed in literature, can indeed explain the experimental findings.

Mathematical models are also a practical tool for the optimization of the properties of (CaP) scaffolds and the tissue engineering process in general. Byrne et al. [8] showed that scaffolds could be tailored for the site of implantation, which is characterized by specific loading conditions. In a low loading environment, a highly porous and stiff scaffold with medium dissolution rate would give the greatest amount of bone. In a high loading environment, however, a low initial porosity and rate of dissolution are necessary to maintain the mechanical and structural integrity of the bone-scaffold system [8]. Checa et al. [12] investigated the effect of cell seeding density on the bone formation process. They found that a reduction in the initial MSC seeding density increased the amount of bone formation since the vessels could more easily penetrate the construct ensuring the supply of oxygen and nutrients. The model of Carlier et al. [11] is able to define the optimal scaffold properties (in terms of Ca^{2+} release) for different initial cell seeding conditions. Moreover, the model can be used to determine the optimal scaffold properties for different cell types (e.g. hPDC, hBMSC) since these cell types are characterized by different proliferation and differentiation parameters. This optimal dissolution rate could be an input parameter for the model of Bohner et al. [6] to determine the optimized microstructural properties of the CaP scaffold.

Besides the optimization of scaffold properties or seeding protocols, mathematical modeling allows for an *in silico* screening of novel biomaterials based on biomaterial characteristics encompassed in the model (such as calcium release rate in Carlier et al. [11]) thereby increasing the initial quality of the biomaterials selected for *in vivo* experimentation and reducing the number of false positive or negative results. Moreover, mathematical modeling can help to design and test possible treatment strategies. Peiffer et al. [33] used a hybrid bioregulatory model of angiogenesis during fracture healing to investigate the effect of vascular endothelial growth factor (VEGF) on the healing of MMP9 deficient fractures. They convincingly show that a treatment comprising daily bolus injections of VEGF is not as efficient as using a slow-release VEGF carrier. Similarly, Geris et al. [15] used an *in silico* technique to investigate the effect of MSC injection in an atrophic non-union model. They show that after the injection of the cell transplant in the callus region, the amount of bone was predicted to increase whereas the amount of fibrous tissue was predicted to decrease. The amount of soft tissue was however strongly dependent on the exact location of injection of the cell transplant with excentral injection leading to unicortical bridging. The model of Carlier et al. [11] shows that insufficient cell seeding on CaP scaffolds may lead to impaired bone formation due to the very high Ca^{2+} concentration that negatively influences cellular proliferation and differentiation. The *in silico* treatment strategy of exponentially reducing the calcium release after implantation was found to lead to bone formation. The controlled ad hoc reduction of calcium release after implantation is not feasible in reality. However, owing to cellular attachment and protein adsorption, the theoretical release rates which are generally determined in acellular dissolution experiments most likely do not correspond to the actual release rates *in vivo*.

Mathematical models are often less time consuming than experimental research. Due to the enormous increase in computational power, both on a personal workstation as in high performance computing facilities, computer simulations can be used to model and optimize biological processes. In the model of Carlier et al. [11] this time gain is quite dramatic, simulating the process of bone formation that occurs over 90 days in only a few minutes. Also, experimental research is often much more expensive than mathematical modeling. Simple mathematical models can be easily simulated on a personal workstation whereas wet lab facilities require specific laboratories and equipment. Moreover, the cost of specific biological components and transgenic animals can be very significant.

3.2 *... to Experiments ...*

Although computational modeling has many advantages, it will never fully replace experimental research. As already mentioned, mathematical models can help experimental research in several ways. Firstly, mathematical models ask fundamental questions and provoke discussion. Secondly, mathematical models contribute to the general knowledge of the biological processes. Thirdly, mathematical models can be used to guide experimental design. But the experimental research is also invaluable for mathematical modeling. Experimental research is necessary to establish the fundamental knowledge on the biological processes and allows determining the important parameters and their respective parameter values. Experimental research also plays a key role in the validation of mathematical models.

As already mentioned in the previous section, there is a strong need for more quantitative data. Extensive quantification of *in vitro* and *in vivo* measurements and characterization of (CaP) scaffold properties would not only allow a more accurate determination of the model parameter values but also a more complete validation and enhancement of the model predictions. However, experimental research is often still qualitative. Moreover, the experimental measurements do not necessarily correspond to the data that are needed in the modeling framework. It is therefore imperative that *in vivo* and *in vitro* experiments are specifically designed and set-up to match to modeling conditions in order to further validate and improve the model's predictions.

As an essential part of the integrative approach that Carlier et al. [11] use to investigate the effect of Ca^{2+} on the bone forming capacity of CaP scaffolds, specific *in vitro* experiments were performed to determine the effect of Ca^{2+} on the proliferation of MSCs and osteoblasts. In short, cells were expanded in a monolayer using growth medium. Upon confluence, human periosteal derived cells (hPDCs) were re-plated and synchronized. Freshly prepared Ca^{2+} supplemented growth media were then added to the cell cultures and incubated for 1, 3, 7, 14, 21 and 28 days before being harvested for analysis. At each time point the DNA content was quantified. The data measured at 7 days ware assumed to be representative of MSC proliferation, whereas the data measured at 28 days were assumed to be representative of cells further down the osteoblastic lineage. A least-square fitting through the experimental data determined the parameters that characterize the influence of calcium on the proliferation of MSCs and osteoblasts.

Another example of this challenge in experimental research is the determination of the dissolution rate of CaP scaffolds. As shown by Carlier et al. [11], this property has an important effect on the final amount of bone formation and should as such be thoroughly characterized. However, the degradation rate is influenced by many scaffold characteristics (e.g. micro- and macrostructure, the material composition, specific surface area) and testing conditions (e.g. temperature, composition of dissolution medium, pH, specific surface area to medium ratio). Currently dissolution tests still lack standardization [22] and often the (CaP) scaffolds are not completely characterized, making it very difficult to compare the results of different studies found in literature. Impens et al. [22] show for example that perfusion tests result in a higher dissolution rate when compared to bath shaking tests due to the easier entrance of the fluid flow inside these scaffold. Moreover, these *in vitro* tests do not take the influence of protein adsorption or osteoclastic activity after implantation into account. From the above it is clear that there is still a long way to go and that specific experiments should be designed that resemble the *in vivo* conditions as close as possible.

3.3 ... and Back

The multidisciplinary problem of optimizing scaffold architecture and seeding protocols for bone tissue engineering strategies requires an integrative approach. This strategy uses mathematical modeling to explain a mechanism of biomaterial-cell interactions in combination with experimental research to provide data for the determination of the model parameters as well as the validation of the model [5]. Moreover, this process is inherently iterative, where new experimental results can be fed to the model and thorough model analysis can lead to new research hypotheses.

4 Prospects

Most of the current models look either at mechanoregulatory or bioregulatory stimuli, depending on the specific research question that is being answered. In the future, however, these models could be combined to further improve the predictive capabilities of the model. Another issue is the specific scale at which most models are created. Some models look in more detail at a small scale (e.g. [11]) while others look at a larger scale [8, 15]. The problem of bone regeneration inside (CaP) scaffolds is however regulated by countless biochemical and mechanical factors across multiple organizational scales. The time scales of these individual events range from seconds for phosphorylation events to hours for mRNA transcription to weeks for tissue formation and remodeling processes [26]. The spatial scales vary from nanometers at the molecular level to millimeters at the tissue level and meters at the level of the organism [26, 30]. As such, one can conclude that the bone regeneration process is a multiscale problem and should be studied and modeled accordingly. Some attempts have already been made like Sanz-Herrera et al. [38] who use a multiscale modeling approach to determine the role of the scaffold microarchitecture in bone tissue regeneration. Besides some localized activities, coordinated efforts should also focus on the integration of models at different biological scales [26]. Liu et al. [26] propose for example an object-oriented module-based computational integration strategy to link currently available models of different methodologies (algebraic equations, PDEs, AB). In this way the computational infrastructure effectively integrates multiple modules by coordinating their connectivity and data exchange. Not only does such a platform allow the straightforward combination of existing mathematical models, it is also intrinsically a multiscale modeling environment thereby approaching the true multiscale nature of biological processes.

As already pinpointed in the previous section, quantitative data are crucial for mathematical models to reach their true potential. Thus *in vitro* or *in vivo* experiments should be designed so that they enable quantification. The highly controllable and quantifiable environment is a major advantage of *in vitro* set-ups [18]. However, the conclusions should be carefully translated to the actual *in vivo* environment since the cells and tissues are isolated from their natural environment. The use of *in vivo* models has the advantage of resembling the reality but quantification will be more challenging. Moreover, as mathematical models predict the dynamics at different scales (e.g. molecular, cellular and tissue) as a function of time and space, there is a need for temporal and spatial experimental data. A possible strategy is the use of imaging techniques (e.g. micro-computed tomography) that allow non-invasively monitoring and quantification of the *in vivo* dynamics.

5 Conclusion

This chapter discussed the biology of bone regeneration in CaP scaffolds and the related modeling efforts. A number of advantages of mathematical modeling were indicated and illustrated by examples of the bone tissue engineering field. It is clear that only a true integrative approach, that combines mathematical modeling with experimental research will help to further elucidate the biological process of bone regeneration inside CaP scaffolds. The integrative strategy is necessary during both the development of the model (determination of parameter values) and the model validation phase (comparison of the model predictions to experimental findings). Building this bridge between different disciplines requires a lot of effort but it is the only way to truly obtain predictive models that can be used to advance the research in the bone tissue engineering field.

Acknowledgements Aurélie Carlier is a PhD fellow of the Research Foundation Flanders (FWO-Vlaanderen). The work is part of Prometheus, the Leuven Research and Development Division of Skeletal Tissue Engineering of that Katholieke Universiteit Leuven: www.kuleuven.be/Prometheus.

Appendix

The equations contain the following model parameters:

$$J(t) = J_{in} \cdot \frac{Ca(t)}{H_{Ca4} + Ca(t)}$$

$$A_m(t) = \frac{A_{m0} \cdot m(t)}{K_m^2 + m(t)^2}$$

$$\beta_{cm}(t) = \frac{a_{cm}}{c_{cm}} \cdot \exp\left(-\frac{1}{2} \cdot \left(\frac{Ca(t) - b_{cm}}{c_{cm}}\right)^2\right)$$

$$F_1(t) = \frac{Y_{11} \cdot g_b(t)^6}{H_{11}^6 + g_b(t)^6} \cdot F_{11} \cdot \exp\left(-\frac{1}{2} \cdot (Ca(t) - F_{12})^2\right)$$

$$A_b(t) = \frac{A_{b0} \cdot m(t)}{K_b^2 + m(t)^2}$$

$$\beta_{cb}(t) = \frac{a_{cb}}{c_{cb}} \cdot \exp\left(-\frac{1}{2} \cdot \left(\frac{Ca(t) - b_{cb}}{c_{cb}}\right)^2\right)$$

$$E_{gb}(t) = \frac{G_{gb} \cdot g_b(t)}{H_{gb} + g_b(t)}$$

$$R(t) = \left|c_m(t) - c_m(t - t_3)\right| \cdot \frac{G_{con} \cdot g_b(t)}{H_{con} + g_b(t)}$$

The following scaling factors were chosen for the non-dimensionalization of the model variables:

$$\widetilde{t} = \frac{t}{T}, \qquad \widetilde{c_m} = \frac{c_m}{c_0}, \qquad \widetilde{c_b} = \frac{c_b}{c_0}, \qquad \widetilde{m} = \frac{m}{m_0}$$

$$\widetilde{b} = \frac{b}{m_0}, \qquad \widetilde{g_b} = \frac{g_b}{g_0}, \qquad \widetilde{Ca} = \frac{Ca}{Ca_0}$$

The time $T = 1$ day was considered to be a representative unit time for the process under study (similar to fracture healing models e.g. Geris et al. [50]). Representative concentrations for the collagen content ($m_0 = 0.1$ g/ml) and growth factors ($g_0 = 100$ ng/ml) are adopted from Geris et al. [50]. A typical value for the cell density ($c_0 = 10^6$ cells/ml) is derived from Bailón-Plaza and van der Meulen [48]. The

Table 1 Non-dimensionalized parameter values of the presented model (tildes are omitted for simplicity)

Parameter	Nominal value	Source
MSCs		
α_m	1	Bailón-Plaza et al. [48]
A_{m0}	0.85	Bailón-Plaza et al. [48]
K_m	0.1	Bailón-Plaza et al. [48]
a_{cm}	5.98	measured
b_{cm}	1.67	measured
c_{cm}	3.33	measured
Y_{11}	10	Bailón-Plaza et al. [48]
H_{11}	14	Bailón-Plaza et al. [48]
F_{11}	8	Dvorak et al. [13]
F_{12}	1.5	Dvorak et al. [13]
d_{cm}	1.5	estimated
Osteoblasts		
A_{b0}	0.202	Bailón-Plaza et al. [48]
K_b	0.1	Bailón-Plaza et al. [48]
α_b	1	Bailón-Plaza et al. [48]
a_{cb}	41.82	measured
b_{cb}	5.06	measured
c_{cb}	1.9	measured
d_b	0.1	Bailón-Plaza et al. [48]
γ	7	measured
Collagen matrix		
P_{bs}	0.18	Yuan et al. [53]
κ_b	1	Bailón-Plaza et al. [48]
Mineral matrix		
δ	0.05	estimated
P_{bb}	0.0398	Yuan et al. [53]
κ_{bb}	1	Bailón-Plaza et al. [48]
m_{thres}	0.85	estimated

scaling factor for the calcium concentration was assumed to be equal to the extra-cellular calcium concentration ($Ca_0 = 1$ mM). An overview of the model parameter values and the initial variable values is given in Table 1 and Table 2 respectively.

The model parameters were non-dimensionalized as follows (the tildes represent the non-dimensional parameters):

Table 1 (Continued)

Parameter	Nominal value	Source
Calcium		
σ	10	estimated
Ca_∞	50	Maeno et al. [51]
J_{in}	750	estimated
H_{Ca4}	0.01	estimated
d_{ca}	100	estimated
Growth factors		
G_{gb}	350	Geris et al. [50]
H_{gb}	1	Geris et al. [50]
G_{con}	1	estimated
H_{con}	0.001	estimated
d_{gb}	75	Geris et al. [50]

Table 2
Non-dimensionalized initial variable values of the presented model

Variable	Nominal value	Source
c_{m0}	1	Eyckmans et al. [49]
c_{b0}	0	estimated
m_0	0.01	Liu et al. [52]
b_0	0	estimated
g_{b0}	15	Liu et al. [27]
ca_0	1	estimated

$$\widetilde{P_{bs}} = \frac{P_{bs}.c_0.T}{m_0}, \qquad \widetilde{\kappa_b} = \kappa_b.m_0, \qquad \widetilde{A_{m0}} = \frac{A_{m0}.T}{m_0},$$

$$\widetilde{K_m} = \frac{K_m}{m_0}, \qquad \widetilde{a_{cm}} = \frac{a_{cm}}{Ca_0}, \qquad \widetilde{b_{cm}} = \frac{b_{cm}}{Ca_0},$$

$$\widetilde{c_{cm}} = \frac{c_{cm}}{Ca_0}, \qquad \widetilde{\alpha_m} = \alpha_m.c_0, \qquad \widetilde{H_{11}} = \frac{H_{11}}{g_0},$$

$$\widetilde{Y_{11}} = Y_{11}.T, \qquad \widetilde{G_{gb}} = \frac{G_{gb}.T.c_0}{g_0}, \qquad \widetilde{H_{gb}} = \frac{H_{gb}}{g_0},$$

$$\widetilde{d_{gb}} = d_{gb}.T, \qquad \widetilde{A_{b0}} = \frac{A_{b0}.T}{m_0}, \qquad \widetilde{K_b} = \frac{K_b}{m_0}, \qquad \widetilde{a_{cb}} = \frac{a_{cb}}{Ca_0},$$

$$\widetilde{b_{cb}} = \frac{b_{cb}}{Ca_0}, \qquad \widetilde{c_{cb}} = \frac{c_{cb}}{Ca_0}, \qquad \widetilde{\alpha_b} = \alpha_b.c_0,$$

$$\widetilde{d_b} = d_b.T, \qquad \widetilde{P_{bb}} = \frac{P_{bb}.c_0.T}{m_0}, \qquad \widetilde{\kappa_{bb}} = \kappa_{bb}.m_0,$$

$$\tilde{\sigma} = \sigma.T, \qquad \widetilde{Ca_\infty} = \frac{Ca_\infty}{Ca_0}, \qquad \widetilde{J_{leaky}} = \frac{J_{leaky}.T.c_0}{Ca_0},$$

$$\widetilde{H_{ca4}} = \frac{H_{ca4}}{Ca_0}, \qquad \widetilde{d_{Ca}} = d_{Ca}.T.c_0, \qquad \widetilde{F_{11}} = F_{11}, \qquad \widetilde{F_{12}} = F_{12},$$

$$\widetilde{G_{con}} = G_{con}.c_0, \qquad \widetilde{H_{con}} = \frac{H_{con}}{g_0}, \qquad \widetilde{d_{cm}} = d_{cm}.T.m_0$$

References

1. Barrère F, van Blitterswijk C, de Groot K (2006) Bone regeneration: molecular and cellular interactions with calcium phosphate ceramic. Int J Nanomed 1:317–332
2. Barrère F, van der Valk C, Dalmeijer R, Meijer G, van Blitterswijk C, de Groot K, Layrolle P (2003) Osteogenecity of octacalcium phosphate coatings applied on porous metal implants. J Biomed Mater Res, Part A 66:779–788
3. Beck Jr. GR Knecht N (2003) Osteopontin regulation by inorganic phosphate is ERK1/2-, protein kinase C-, and proteasome-dependent. J Biol Chem 278:41921–41929
4. Bhandari M, Jain AK (2009) Bone stimulators: beyond the black box. Indian J Orthop 43:109–110
5. Bohner M, Loosli Y, Baroud G, Lacroix D (2011) Commentary: deciphering the link between architecture and biological response in a bone graft substitute. Acta Biomater 7:478–484
6. Bohner M, Baumgart F (2004) Theoretical model to determine the effects of geometrical factors on the resorption of calcium phosphate bone substitutes. Biomaterials 25:3569–3582
7. Bootman M, Young K, Young J, Moreton R, Berridge M (1996) Extracellular calcium concentration controls the frequency of intracellular calcium spiking independently of inositol 1, 4,5-triphosphate production in hela cells. Biochem J 314:347–354
8. Byrne DP, Lacroix D, Planell JA, Kelly DJ, Prendergast PJ (2007) Simulation of tissue differentiation in a scaffold as a function of porosity, Young's modulus and dissolution rate: application of mechanobiological models in tissue engineering. Biomaterials 28:5544–5554
9. Chai YC, Roberts SJ, Schrooten J, Luyten FP (2011) Probing the osteoinductive effect of calcium phosphate by using an in vitro biomimetic model. Tissue Eng A 17(7–8):1083–1097
10. Chang Y, Stanford C, Keller J (2000) Calcium and phosphate supplementation promotes bone cell mineralization: implications for hydroxyapatite-enhanced bone formation. J Biomed Mater Res 52:240–278
11. Carlier A, Chai Y, Moesen M, Theys T, Schrooten J, Van Oosterwyck H, Geris L (2011) Designing optimal calcium phosphate scaffold-cell combinations using an integrative model based approach. Acta Biomater 7:3573–3585
12. Checa S, Prendergast PJ (2010) Effect of cell seeding and mechanical loading on vascularization and tissue formation inside a scaffold: a mechano-biological model using a lattice approach to simulate cell activity. J Biomech 43:961–968
13. Dvorak M, Siddiqua A, Ward D, Carter D, Dallas S, Nemeth E, Riccardi D (2004) Physiological changes in extracellular calcium concentration directly control osteoblast function in the absence of calciotropic hormones. Proc Natl Acad Sci USA 101:5140–5145
14. Eyckmans J, Roberts S, Schrooten J, Luyten F (2010) A clinically relevant model of osteoinduction: a process requiring calcium phosphate and BMP/Wnt signaling. J Cell Mol Med 14:1845–1856
15. Geris L, Reed AAC, Vander Sloten J, Simpson AHRW, Van Oosterwyck H (2010) Occurrence and treatment of bone atrophic non-unions investigated by an integrative approach. PLoS Comput Biol 6(9):e1000915. doi:10.1371/journal.pcbi.1000915

16. Geris L, Gerisch A Schugart RC (2010) Mathematical modeling in wound healing, bone regeneration and tissue engineering. Acta Biotheor 58:355–367
17. Geris L, Schugart RC, Van Oosterwyck H (2010) In silico design of treatment strategies in wound healing and bone fracture healing. Philos Trans R Soc Lond A 368:2683–2706
18. Geris L, Vander Sloten J, Van Oosterwyck H (2009) In silico biology of bone modelling and remodelling: regeneration. Philos Trans R Soc, Math Phys Eng Sci 367:2031–2053
19. Habibovic P, de Groot K (2007) Osteoinductive biomaterials—properties and relevance in bone repair. J Tissue Eng Regen Med 1:25–32
20. Hanawa T, Kamiura Y, Yamamoto S, Kohgo T, Amemiya A, Ukai H et al (1997) Early bone formation around calcium-ion-implanted titanium inserted into rat tibia. J Biomed Mater Res 36:131–135
21. Hartman E, Vehof J, Spauwen P, Jansen J (2005) Ectopic bone formation in rats: the importance of the carrier. Biomaterials 26:1829–1835
22. Impens S, Schelstraete R, Mullens S, Thijs I, Luyten J, Schrooten J (2008) scaffolds for bone tissue engineering. In: vitro dissolution behavior of custom made CaP. Key eng mater, vol 20, pp 7–10
23. Julien M, Khoshniat S, Lacreusette A, Gatius M, Bozec A, Wagner EF et al (2009) Phosphate-dependent regulation of MGP in osteoblasts: role of ERK1/2 and Fra-1. J Bone Miner Res 24:1856–1868
24. Lacroix D, Planell JA, Prendergast PJ (2009) Computer-aided design and finite-element modelling of biomaterial scaffold for bone tissue engineering. Philos Trans R Soc Lond A 367:1993–2009
25. Langer R, Vacanti JP (1993) Tissue engineering. Science 260(5510):920–926
26. Liu G, Qutub A, Vempati P, Mac Gabhann F, Popel AS (2011) Module-based multiscale simulation of angiogenesis in skeletal muscle. Theor Biol Med Model 8:6
27. Liu YK, Lu QZ, Pei R, Ji HJ, Zhou GS, Zhao XL et al (2009) The effect of extracellular calcium and inorganic phosphate on the growth and osteogenic differentiation of mesenchymal stem cells in vitro: implication for bone tissue engineering. Biomed Mater 4:025004
28. Liu YK, Wang GC, Cai YR, Ji HJ, Zhou GS, Zhao XL, Tang RK, Zhang M (2008) In vitro effects of nanophase hydroxyapatite particles on proliferation and osteogenic differentiation of bone marrow-derived mesenchymal stem cells. J Biomed Mater Res, Part A 90(4):1083–1091
29. Massa A (2007) The merging field of regenerative medicine. MMG 445 Basic Biotech eJournal 3:137–143
30. Meier-Schellersheim M, Fraser I, Klauschen F (2009) Multiscale modeling for biologists. WIREs Syst Biol Med 1:4–14
31. Milan JL, Planell JA, Lacroix D (2010) Simulation of bone tissue formation within a porous scaffold under dynamic compression. Biomech Model Mechanobiol 9:583–596
32. Murshed M, Harmey D, Millan JL, McKee MD, Karsenty G (2005) Unique coexpression in osteoblasts of broadly expressed genes accounts for the spatial restriction of ECM mineralization to bone. Genes Dev 19:1093–1104
33. Peiffer V, Gerisch A, Vandepitte D, Van Oosterwyck H, Geris L (2011) A hybrid bioregulatory model of angiogenesis during bone fracture healing. Biomech Model Mechanobiol 10:383–395
34. Pioletti D, Takei H, Lin T, Van Landuyt P, Ma Q, Kwon S, Sung KL (2000) The effects of calcium phosphate cement particles on osteoblast functions. Biomaterials 21:1103–1114
35. Ripamonti U (1996) Osteoinduction in porous hydroxyapatite implanted in heterotopic sites of different animal models. Biomaterials 17:31–35
36. Roberts SJ, Geris L, Kerckhofs G, Desmet E, Schrooten J, Luyten F (2011) The combined bone forming capacity of human periosteal derived cells and calcium phosphates. Biomaterials 32:4393–4405
37. Sanz-Herrera JA, Garcia-Aznar JM, Doblare M (2008) A mathematical model for bone tissue regeneration inside a specific type of scaffold. Biomech Model Mechanobiol 7:355–366
38. Sanz-Herrera JA, García-Aznar JM, Doblaré M (2008) Micro-macro numerical modeling of bone regeneration in tissue engineering. Comput Methods Appl Mech Eng 197:3092–3107

39. Sengers BG, Taylor M, Please C, Oreffo RO (2007) Computational modeling of cell spreading and tissue regeneration in porous scaffolds. Biomaterials 28:1926–1940
40. Shelton RM, Rasmussen AC, Davies JE (1988) Protein adsorption at the interface between charged polymer substrata and migrating osteoblasts. Biomaterials 9:24–29
41. Stein GS, Lian JB, Stein JL, van Wijnen AJ, Frenkel B, Monteccino M (1996) Mechanisms regulating osteoblast proliferation and differentiation. In: Bilezikian JP, Raisz LG, Rodan GA (eds) Principles of bone biology. Academic Press, California, pp 69–87
42. Stops AJF, Heraty KB, Browne M, O'Brien FJ, McHugh PE (2010) A prediction of cell differentiation and proliferation within a collagen-glycosaminoglycan scaffold subjected to mechanical strain and perfusive fluid flow. J Biomech 43(4):618–626
43. Sun S, Liu Y, Lipsky S, Cho M (2007) Physical manipulation of calcium oscillations facilitates osteodifferentiation of human mesenchymal stem cells. FASEB J 21:1472–1480
44. Titorencu I, Jinga V, Constantinescu E, Gafencu A, Ciohodaru C, Manolescu I et al (2007) Proliferation, differentiation and characterization of osteoblasts from human BM mesenchymal stem cells. Cytotherapy 9:682–696
45. van der Meulen MC, Huiskes R (2002) Why mechanobiology? A survey article. J Biomech 35:401–414
46. Yuan H, van Blitterswijk C, de Groot K, de Bruijn J (2006) A comparison of bone formation in biphasic calcium phosphate and hydroxyapatite implanted in muscle and bone of dogs at different time periods. J Biomed Mater Res, Part A 78:130–147
47. Zhou GS, Su ZY, Cai YR, Liu YK, Dai LC, Tang RK, Zhang M (2007) Different effects of nanophase and conventional hydroxyapatite thin films on attachment, proliferation and osteogenic differentiation of bone marrow derived mesenchymal stem cells. Biomed Mater Eng 17:387–395
48. Bailón-Plaza A, van der Meulen M (2001) A mathematical framework to study the effects of growth factor influences on fracture healing. J Theor Biol 212:191–209
49. Eyckmans J, Roberts S, Schrooten J, Luyten F (2010) A clinically relevant model of osteoinduction: a process requiring calcium phosphate and BMP/Wnt signaling. J Cell Mol Med 14:1845–1856
50. Geris L, Gerisch A, Vander Sloten J, Weiner R, Van Oosterwyck H (2008) Angiogenesis in bone fracture healing: A bioregulatory model. J Theor Biol 251:137–158
51. Maeno S, Niki Y, Matsumoto H, Morioka H, Yatabe T, Funayama A et al (2005) The effect of calcium ion concentration on osteoblast viability, proliferation and differentiation in monolayer and 3D culture. Biomaterials 26:4847–4855
52. Liu Y, Lu Q, Pei R, Ji H, Zhou G, Zhao X et al (2009) The effect of extracellular calcium and inorganic phosphate on the growth and osteogenic differentiation of mesenchymal stem cells in vitro: implication for bone tissue engineering. Biomed Mater 4(2):025004
53. Yuan H, van Blitterswijk C, de Groot K, de Bruijn J (2006) A comparison of bone formation in biphasic calcium phosphate and hydroxyapatite implanted in muscle and bone of dogs at different time periods. J Biomed Mater Res, Part A 78:130–417

Constitutive Effects of Hydrolytic Degradation in Electro-Spun Polyester-Urethane Scaffolds for Soft Tissue Regeneration

Hugo Krynauw, Lucie Bruchmüller, Deon Bezuidenhout, Peter Zilla, and Thomas Franz

Abstract In tissue regenerative implants, porosity allowing the ingrowth of cells and tissue is a key factor for the long-term success. While vital for healing and tissue regeneration, the use of highly porous structures may adversely affect the mechanical properties of the scaffold, in particular when viscoelastic polymeric materials are used. In the case of biodegradable scaffold materials, the effect of the degradation process on mechanical and structural properties of the scaffold is yet another aspect to be considered. Both tissue ingrowth and biodegradation are concurrent transient processes which change the mechanical and structural properties of the implanted device over time. Ingrowth of cells and tissue typically results in an increase in structural stiffness whereas scaffold degradation leads to loss of mechanical properties and potentially to structural disintegration. The aim of the research presented in this chapter was the investigation of the change of mechanical properties of a biodegradable, electro-spun polyester-urethane scaffold for soft tissue regeneration during hydrolytic degradation and the development of a constitutive model that is suitable for capturing these changes.

1 Introduction

Tissue engineering and tissue regeneration are prominent tools in regenerative medicine for the treatment of diseases and injuries [1, 2]. Biodegradable scaffolds have been used and have shown promises for the future of tissue regenerative pros-

H. Krynauw (✉) · L. Bruchmüller · D. Bezuidenhout · P. Zilla · T. Franz
Cardiovascular Research Unit, Chris Barnard Division of Cardiothoracic Surgery,
University of Cape Town, Cape Town, South Africa
e-mail: kryhug001@myuct.ac.za

T. Franz
Centre for Research in Computational and Applied Mechanics, University of Cape Town,
Rondebosch, Cape Town, South Africa
e-mail: Thomas.Franz@uct.ac.za

T. Franz
Research Office, University of Cape Town, Mowbray, Observatory, Cape Town, South Africa

P.R. Fernandes, P.J. Bártolo (eds.), *Tissue Engineering*,
Computational Methods in Applied Sciences 31, DOI 10.1007/978-94-007-7073-7_3,
© Springer Science+Business Media Dordrecht 2014

thesis. Implants need to be designed such that their behaviour matches, in the ideal case both biologically and mechanically, that of the organ or tissue to be replaced in its healthy state [1]. In the treatment of cardiovascular diseases, examples of regenerative medicine include tissue regenerative small diameter vascular grafts. In such grafts, porosity allowing the ingrowth of cells and tissue is a key factor for the long-term success [3]. Porous scaffolds have been manufactured in different ways including phase inversion and porogen extraction [4, 5] salt leaching [6], gas foaming [7], extrusion-phase-inversion [8], thermally induced phase separation [9] and electro-spinning [10–12].

While imperative for healing and tissue regeneration, porosity may adversely affect the structural properties of the vascular scaffold, in particular when viscoelastic polymeric materials are used. This increases the complexity of the structural design of tissue regenerative vascular scaffolds which should, ideally, mimic non-linear elastic mechanics of the vascular soft tissue [13, 14]. The desired structural properties may not be attainable with prostheses consisting of a single material but demand a more complex structure comprising multiple components and/or materials. Due to the intricacy of the structural design process, computational methods have been employed for the development and optimisation of cardiovascular implants [15–17]. The numerical prediction of structural properties of grafts requires the knowledge of the mechanical properties of the scaffold materials. Based on experimentally determined material properties, constitutive models can be used, or developed if required, for a realistic computational representation of the material's mechanics. Constitutive models of porous structures, such as foams, can be based at microscopic and macroscopic scale, respectively. At microscopic level, a constitutive model utilises the bulk properties of the porous material combined with representation of the microscopic geometrical features. This approach requires typically extensive computational resources and may not be feasible for large ranges between microscopic and macroscopic dimensions of the physical problem. Alternatively, a constitutive model may utilise the mechanical properties of the porous material at macroscopic level, e.g. of a foam. In this 'smearing' approach, the porous structure is numerically treated as a homogeneous material without the need to represent microscopic geometrical features [16, 18].

The optimal design of tissue regenerative vascular prostheses, thus, needs to consider the mechanical properties of the initial scaffold as well as effects of biodegradation, and healing, on the structural mechanics of the implant. Consequently, detailed knowledge is required of the mechanical effects of scaffold degradation.

The mechanical characterisation of biodegradable polymeric materials used for tissue regenerative medical implants such as vascular grafts, has received attention from various research groups. Lendlein et al. [19, 20] studied the mechanical bulk properties of a degradable polyester-urethane (DegraPol®) prior to degradation and during degradation, whereas electro-spun polyester-urethane membranes were mechanically characterised by Riboldi et al. [12]. Kwon et al. [21] determined structural and mechanical properties of electro-spun biodegradable co-polyesters. Mechanical properties prior to degradation have also been reported for electro-spun scaffolds using poly(ε-caprolactone) [22], poly(ε-caprolactone)/collagen [23] and poly(ε-caprolactone)/poly-lactic acid [24].

The change of mechanical properties associated with degradation has been studied for various biodegradable polymers. Raghunath et al. [25] characterised solid sheets of biodegradable polyhedral oligomeric silsesquioxane modified poly(caprolactone/carbonate) urethane/urea during accelerated *in vitro* degradation of up to eight weeks. Kang et al. [26] studied the *in vitro* degradation of a porous poly(l-lactic acid)/β-tricalcium phosphate scaffold, fabricated by particulate leaching, of up to six weeks and reported the effect on the compressive strength.

While the mechanics of electro-spun degradable scaffolds has been investigated prior to degradation, the information on the effects of the degradation process on the mechanical properties is limited. Lee et al. [23] studied the maintenance of tensile properties of electro-spun poly(ε-caprolactone)/collagen scaffolds subjected to a perfusion bioreactor environment for up to four weeks. Henry et al. [27] mechanically characterised electro-spun meshes of a slow degrading polyester-urethane during hydrolytic *in vitro* degradation of up to 346 days.

We investigated a highly porous, electro-spun structure made from a fast-degrading polyester-urethane. The change of structural and mechanical properties of the scaffold was studied during hydrolytic *in vitro* degradation of up to 34 days. Based on these data, a constitutive model for the scaffold was developed that specifically aims at representing the changes in scaffold mechanical properties due to degradation. This is important as the tissue ingrowth and scaffold degradation occurs simultaneously and scaffold contribution during healing must be tailored to compliment that of the new tissue [28].

2 Effects of Degradation on Mechanical Scaffold Properties

2.1 Scaffold Material

DegraPol® (ab medica S.p.A, Lainate, Italy) is a biodegradable polyester-urethane that consists of poly(3-(R-hydroxybutyrate)-co-(ε-caprolactone))-diol (hard segment) and poly(ε-caprolactone-co-glycolide)-diol (soft segment). Both polymer segments are biodegradable and their degradation products are non-toxic [29]. By using different ratios of hard and soft segment the mechanical properties of the final product can be modulated, whereas by changing the ratio of εcaprolactone to glycolide the degradation characteristics can be modulated. This versatility, combined with the non-toxicity and haemocompatibility makes DegraPol® a promising choice for tissue engineering scaffolds. DegraPol® DP30 has a ε-caprolactone-to-glycolide ratio of 70:30 and a hard-to-soft segment ratio of 40:60 (unpublished data). The electro-spinning solution was prepared by dissolving DegraPol® DP30 in chloroform with a 20 % by weight concentration at room temperature and subsequently sonicating in distilled water at 37 °C for 90 min.

2.2 Scaffold Manufacture and Sample Preparation

Tubular samples were prepared by electro-spinning the DegraPol® solution from a hypodermic needle with a flow rate 1.437 ml/h (SE400B syringe pump, Fresenius, Bad Homburg, Germany) onto a tubular target (hypodermic tubing, Small Parts, Loganport, IN, USA; outer diameter: 5.0 mm) rotating at 400 RPM and bi-directionally translating orthogonal to the needle, over a length of 95 mm at a speed of 2.6 mm/min (custom-made drive mechanism). An electrostatic field of 13 kV between the hypodermic needle and the target (distance: 200 mm) was produced by a custom-made high voltage supply. After completion of the spinning process, the electro-spun structure on the target hypotube was submersed in ethanol for 5 minutes, cut open lengthwise, removed from the mandrel and dried under vacuum (Townson & Mercer Ltd, Stretford, England; room temperature, 90 min). Due to the decreasing wall thickness in the end regions, a section of 10–20 mm was cut off on either end of the electro-spun tube and discarded. The tubular scaffolds were cut into 10 mm wide strips yielding 10×18.5 mm rectangular samples (when unfolded) with the longer edge aligned with rotational direction of the spinning target. Wall thickness, width and length of scaffold samples were measured on macroscopic images captured on a Leica DFC280 stereo microscope using Leica IM500 imaging software (Leica Microsystems GmbH, Wetzlar, Germany), see Fig. 1(a, b). Six thickness measurements were recorded on both length edges of each sample as well as six measurements for sample width. The average wall thickness of the tubular scaffolds was 0.99 ± 0.18 mm.

Scanning electron microscope (SEM) (JEOL JSM5200, JEOL Ltd, Tokyo, Japan, 25 kV) analysis was conducted on samples sputter coated with gold (Polaron SC7640, Quorum Technologies, East Grinstead, England). Figure 1(c–f) shows SEM micrographs of the fibrous structure at various magnifications.

Fibre diameter was measured on $\times 2000$ SEM micrographs (one image per sample, ten measurements per image) with Scion Image for Windows (Scion Corporation, Frederick, USA). Fibre diameter was 6.80 ± 2.96 µm, ranging between 1.73 µm and 16.45 µm. Fibre alignment was analysed by two-dimensional Fast Fourier Transforms (2D FFT) of $\times 200$ SEM micrographs in ImageJ (National Institute of Health, Bethesda, MD, USA). The FFT represents the frequency spectrum of the change in pixel intensity of an image. When fibres are aligned (Fig. 2a), the frequency of pixel intensity change will be greater orthogonal to the fibres than in line with them. By using the ImageJ Oval Profile Plot plug-in (written by William O'Connell), a radial summation of pixel intensity in a circular field on the FFT power spectrum (Fig. 2b) can be presented as the fibre alignment orthogonal to summation angle [11, 30, 31]. By scaling the summation results of all images to the range between 0 and 1, the difference in brightness, contrast and number of fibres per image can be normalised. The fibre alignment of the inner and outer wall surface of the electro-spun scaffolds is illustrated Fig. 3. The graphs indicate predominant alignment of the fibres at an angle of 85 to 90° (the latter value representing the circumferential direction of the electro-spun tube) with a more pro-

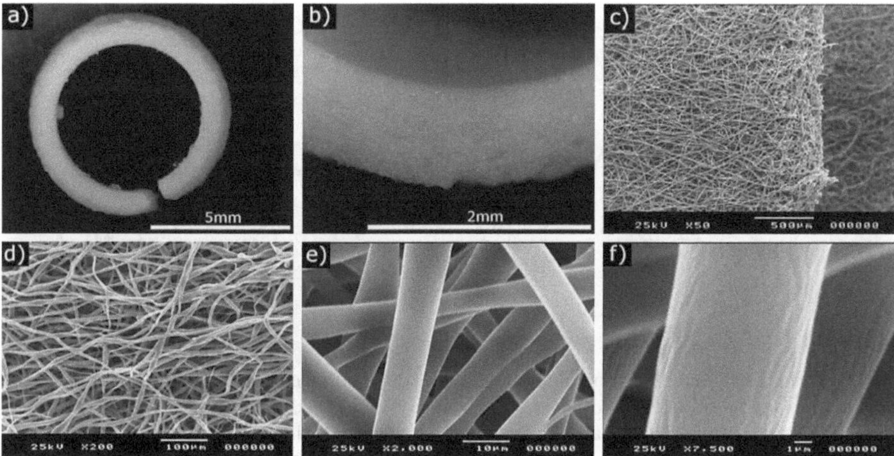

Fig. 1 Gross photographs and micrographs of non-degraded electro-spun scaffold samples. The magnification and scale bar length are provided in parenthesis for each micrograph. (**a**) Low magnification cross-sectional view of sample with longitudinal cut ($\times 1$, 5 mm); (**b**) View of portion of cross-section used for measurement of the wall thickness ($\times 4$, 2 mm); (**c**) Outside surface of scaffold (left portion of image) with cut edge. ($\times 50$, 500 µm); (**d**) View of inner surface used for analysis of fibre alignment ($\times 200$, 100 µm); (**e**) High magnification image used for measurement of fibre thickness ($\times 2000$, 10 µm); (**f**) Section of single fibre of non-degraded sample ($\times 7500$, 1 µm)

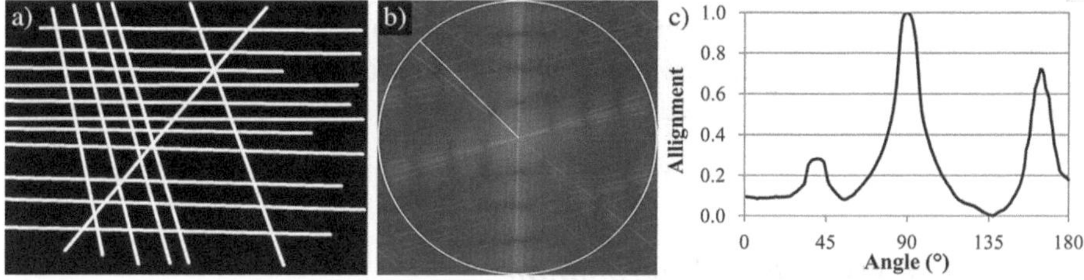

Fig. 2 Example of alignment measure (**a**) Simulated fibre pattern with predominant alignment in one direction; (**b**) FFT power spectrum of example fibre pattern (**a**) showing perimeter of circular summation field and one radial summation line; (**c**) Normalised amount of fibre alignment of fibre pattern in (**a**)

nounced alignment observed on the outer surface compared to the inner surface of the tube.

Scaffold porosity, P, formed by the fibrous network, was calculated from total volume V_T and fibre volume V_F of scaffold samples as $P = 1 - V_F / V_T$. The total volume, i.e. volume of fibres and pores, was determined from wall thickness, width and length of the samples ($n = 3$) measured as described above. The fibre volume, defined as the volume occupied by the fibres excluding all open spaces (pores), was determined by hydrostatic weighing typically employed for density determination. The dry samples were weighed (a) in air and (b) while submerged in ethanol, elim-

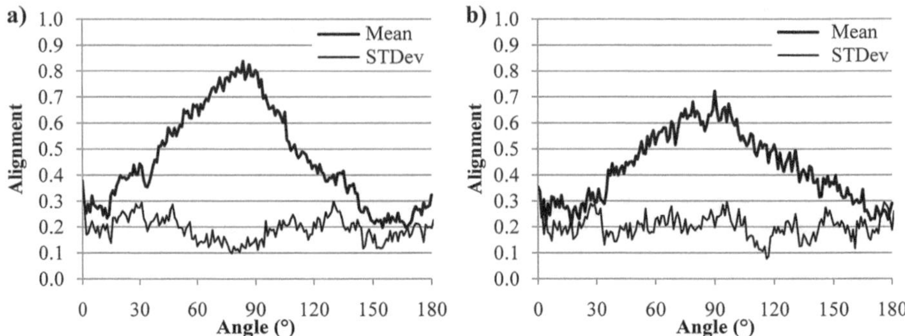

Fig. 3 Normalised amount of fibre alignment on the outer surface (**a**) and inner surface (**b**) of the electro-spun scaffolds versus analysis angle. The analysis angles of 0° and 180° coincide with the longitudinal axis of the target mandrel, and electro-spun tube, whereas the angle of 90° refers to the circumferential direction

inating all air from the scaffold (Adam AAA250L analytical balance with Adam density determination kit, Adam Equipment Inc, Danbury, CT, USA). The difference in mass of the scaffold sample measured in air, $m_{S,air}$, and in ethanol, $m_{S,eth}$, caused by the buoyancy force exerted on the submerged scaffold, equals the mass of the ethanol, m_E, that is displaced by the fibres: $m_E = m_{S,air} - m_{S,eth}$. The volume of the displaced ethanol, V_E, was calculated from the mass, m_E, and the known density of ethanol, ρ_E, as $V_F = V_E = m_E/\rho_E$. Since the volume of the ethanol displaced by the fibres equals the volume of the fibres, the latter is obtained as $V_F = V_E$. The scaffold porosity was determined to be 80 ± 2 %.

2.3 In Vitro Hydrolytic Degradation

For *in vitro* hydrolytic degradation, single samples were placed in a container with 2 ml distilled water and kept at 37 °C (incubator, Scientific Engineering, Johannesburg, South Africa) for degradation time periods of $T = 5, 10, 14, 18, 22, 26, 30$ and 34 days ($n = 5$ samples at each time point). An additional time point of $T = 0$ days refers to non-degraded reference samples. Since the polymer is fast-degrading, non-degraded samples were not soaked, as this would have initiated degradation. After degradation, the samples were removed from water and dried in a vacuum (Townson & Mercer Ltd, Stretford, England; room temperature, 90 min). The pH of the degradation fluid, measured for three samples twice a week (Jenway pH meter 3320, Bibby Scientific Limited, Staffordshire, UK), was 7.2 ± 0.1 at the start of degradation, dropped to 5.9 ± 0.2 at $T = 6$ days and remained at this level ending at 5.7 ± 0.4 at $T = 34$ days.

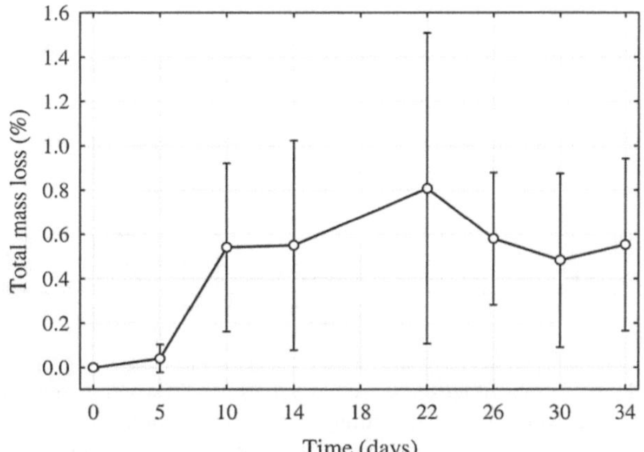

Fig. 4 Cumulative loss of mass, as a percentage of the original sample mass at $T = 0$ days, versus the degradation time

2.4 Physical Characterisation

The scaffold mass (Mettler Toledo XS105S analytical balance, Mettler Toledo, Greifensee, Switzerland) did not change significantly due to degradation. Figure 4 shows the cumulative loss of mass as a percentage of the original sample mass at $T = 0$ days. The largest loss of mass was observed between $T = 5$ and 10 days, increasing from 0.04 ± 0.08 % to 0.54 ± 0.45 %, while it remained at that level thereafter. (For all quantitative data, one-way ANOVA was performed when more than two groups were compared by using Tukey HSD post-hoc analysis with $p < 0.05$ indicating statistical significance. Data are expressed as mean values $\pm$ standard deviation.)

Tensile testing was performed on dry samples at room temperature on an Instron 5544 universal testing machine (Instron, Norwood, USA) using custom made clamps. The width and length of the tensile test samples was 9.69 ± 0.21 mm by 18.47 ± 2.62 mm and the gauge length was 10.40 ± 0.31 mm. The test protocol comprised five pre-cycles (0 to 20 % strain, 20 mm/min crosshead speed, data sampling at 0.1 % strain intervals) and a final extension until complete failure (20 mm/min crosshead speed data sampling at 0.1 % strain intervals). The data recorded were maximum stress σ_{max} and the associated strain ε_{max}, the stress at the upper strain limit of $\varepsilon = 20$ % of each load cycle, $\sigma_{20\,\%,i}$, where i denotes the number of the load cycle with $i = 1$ to 5, and the stress at $\varepsilon = 20$ % of the final loading, $\sigma_{20\,\%,i}$, with $i = 6$. The change in stress associated with cycling was expressed as the ratio, $\sigma_{20\,\%,6}/\sigma_{20\,\%,1}$, of the stress at $\varepsilon = 20$ % during the final and the first loading. The elastic modulus was determined as the slope of the stress-strain curves for the first and the final loading at discrete strain values, $E_{\varepsilon,i}$, where ε refers to the strain value with $\varepsilon = 0, 4, 8, 12, 16$ and 18 %, and i refers to the number of the loading with $i = 1$ and 6. After smoothing of the stress-strain data (moving average filter, half-width: 3), the slope was calculated for the strain range $[\varepsilon - 0.1\,\%, \varepsilon + 0.1\,\%]$ and filtered (moving average filter, half-width: 5). This procedure resulted in elastic modulus values averaged over a range of $[\varepsilon - 0.9\,\%, \varepsilon + 0.9\,\%]$ for each discrete

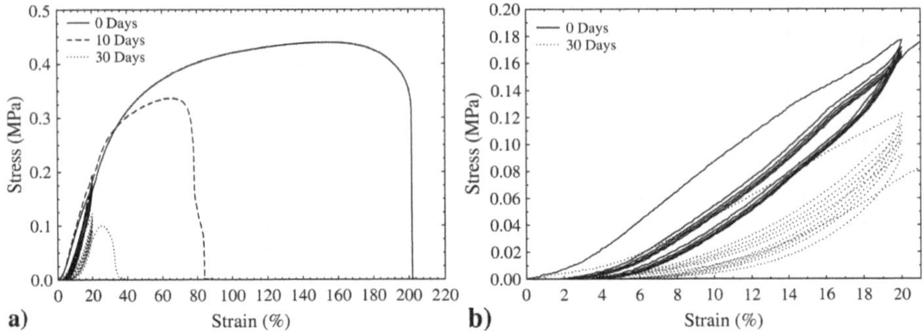

Fig. 5 Graphs of tensile stress, σ, versus tensile strain, ε, representing (**a**) Five initial loading-unloading cycles and final loading until failure of non-degraded sample ($T = 0$ days) and samples degraded for 10 and 30 days, respectively ($T = 10, 30$ days) and (**b**) Close-up of five initial load cycles of non-degraded sample ($T = 0$ days) and samples degraded for 30 days ($T = 30$ days), showing decrease of stress at upper limit of cyclic strain of 20 % with increasing number of cycles. The graph for the sample with $T = 10$ days degradation was omitted to improve clarity of the illustration

value of strain of $\varepsilon = 0, 4, 8, 12, 16$ and 18 %. Stress-strain graphs are presented in Fig. 5(a) for the entire strain range of the tests for samples at degradation time points $T = 0, 10,$ and 30 days and in Fig. 5(b) for limited to the strain range of the load cycles with upper limit of $\varepsilon = 20$ % for degradation time points of $T = 0$ and 30 days.

The maximum stress σ_{max} and associated strain ε_{max} versus degradation time T are illustrated in Fig. 6(a). The stress did not exhibit a change after the first five days of degradation and decreased steadily thereafter. The maximum stress ranged from $\sigma_{max} = 0.52 \pm 0.12$ MPa at $T = 0$ days to $\sigma_{max} = 0.033 \pm 0.028$ MPa after a degradation period of $T = 34$ days. When compared to $T = 0$ days, the decrease in σ_{max} was statistically non-significant up to $T = 14$ days but became statistical significant thereafter. The strain ε_{max} decreased statistically significantly between $T = 0$ days ($\varepsilon_{max} = 176.8 \pm 21.9$ %) and $T = 14$ days ($\varepsilon_{max} = 46.72 \pm 2.35$ %). After $T = 14$ days, the decrease of ε_{max} to the minimum of 24.6 ± 3.0 % at $T = 34$ days occurred at a reduced rate and was non-significant. Figure 6(b) illustrates the stress $\sigma_{20\,\%,i}$ for each repetitive loading event ($i = 1$ to 6) at each degradation time point. Generally, the stress $\sigma_{20\,\%,i}$ decreased with repeated loading. The reduction in stress due to repeated loading (cycling) was less pronounced, and not statistically significant, for the degradation periods up to $T = 18$ days. During the sixth loading, the stress $\sigma_{20\,\%,6}$ reached between 92.4 ± 2.1 % (at $T = 0$ days) and 90.6 ± 1.9 % (at $T = 18$ days) of the initial value at the first loading $\sigma_{20\,\%,1}$, see Fig. 6(c). At degradation of $T = 22$ days and longer, the reduction of $\sigma_{20\,\%,i}$ due to repeated loading increased with degradation time and the ratios $\sigma_{20\,\%,6}/\sigma_{20\,\%,1}$ became statistically significant at $T = 30$ and 34 days ($p = 0.00016$ and 0.00014, respectively, when compared to $T = 18$ days). At $T = 34$ days, the ratio $\sigma_{20\,\%,6}/\sigma_{20\,\%,1}$ was at a minimum of 28.5 ± 16.4 %.

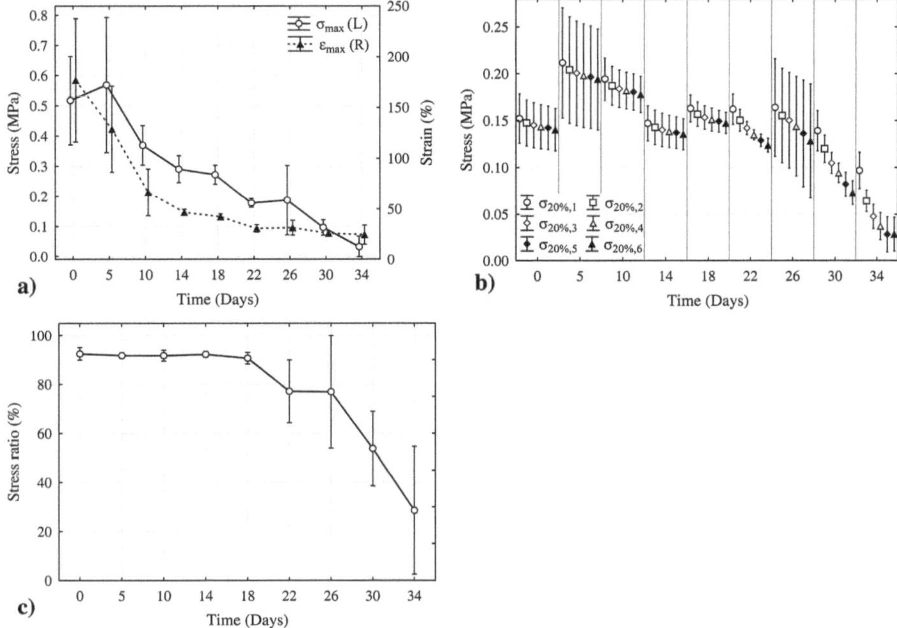

Fig. 6 Characteristic stress and strain data versus degradation time in non-degraded samples ($T = 0$ days) and degraded samples ($T = 5$–34 days): (**a**) Maximum stress, σ_{max}, and corresponding strain, ε_{max}, versus degradation time; (**b**) Stress $\sigma_{20\,\%,i}$ of the five initial loading cycles ($i = 1$ to 5) and the final loading ($i = 6$) versus degradation time; (**c**) Ratio of stress at 20 % strain of final loading to stress at 20 % strain of first cycle, $\sigma_{20\,\%,6}/\sigma_{20\,\%,1}$, versus degradation time

Figure 7 shows the elastic modulus, $E_{\varepsilon,i}$, plotted against strain ε for the first and sixth loading for all degradation time points T. During the first cycle, the elastic modulus exhibited an initial increase with increasing strain but decreased after reaching a maximum between $\varepsilon = 4$ and 8 %, irrespective of the degradation period. However, a steady increase of elastic modulus with increasing strain was typically observed during the sixth loading. Overall, the key values of the elastic modulus for the first loading were $E_{0\,\%,1} = 0.48 \pm 0.35$ MPa, $E_{8\,\%,1} = 0.92 \pm 0.22$ MPa and $E_{18\,\%,1} = 0.67 \pm 0.29$ MPa compared to the values during the sixth loading of $E_{0\,\%,6} = 0.19 \pm 0.19$ MPa, $E_{8\,\%,6} = 0.58 \pm 0.35$ MPa and $E_{18\,\%,6} = 1.1 \pm 0.42$ MPa (all values are grand means over all degradation time points). The maximum elastic modulus during the first and sixth loading, $E_{max,1}$ and $E_{max,6}$, respectively, is provided in Table 1 for scaffolds prior to degradation and for different degradation times points $T = 5$ to 34 days.

2D FFT analysis conducted on SEM micrographs of degraded samples revealed no difference in fibre alignment between the non-degraded and degraded scaffold. The fibre surfaces of scaffold samples after 14 and 34 days degradation prior to mechanical testing are shown in Fig. 8(a, b). Comparison with micrographs in Fig. 1(e, f) indicated that there were no visible differences in surface morphology between degraded and non-degraded fibres. Figure 8(c–f) provides scanning elec-

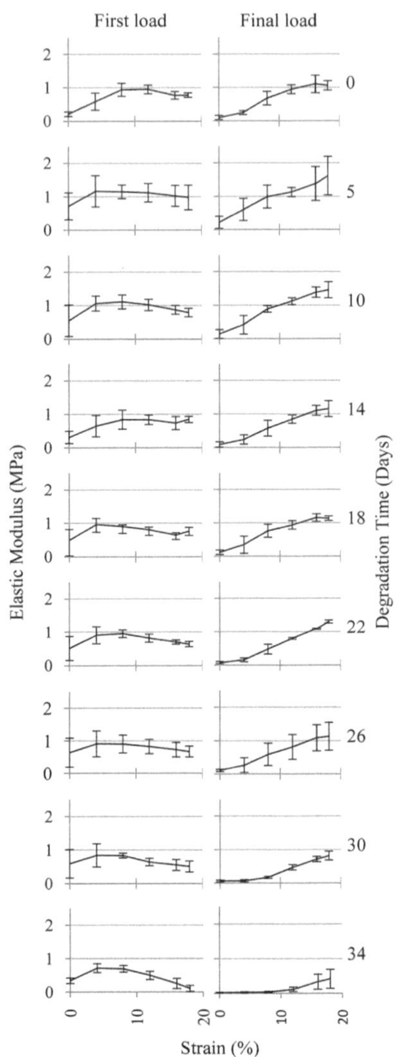

Fig. 7 Elastic modulus of the scaffold versus strain during the first loading ($E_{\varepsilon,1}$) and the final loading ($E_{\varepsilon,6}$) at various degradation time points

tron micrographs of scaffold samples that were degraded for 5 and 26 days, respectively, after mechanical testing to failure.

2.5 Comparative Fibre Alignment Analysis

For comparison purposes, the fibre alignment of the electro-spun scaffold used by Riboldi et al. [12, Figure 1(a)] was determined with the 2D FFT method described above and is presented in Fig. 9.

Table 1 Maximum elastic modulus (mean $\pm$ stdev) of the electro-spun scaffold at the first loading ($E_{\mathrm{max},1}$) and sixth loading ($E_{\mathrm{max},6}$) prior to degradation ($T = 0$ days) and after different times of degradation ($T = 5$ to 34 days)

T (days)	$E_{\mathrm{max},1}$ (MPa)	$E_{\mathrm{max},6}$ (MPa)
0	0.99 ± 0.16	1.14 ± 0.23
5	1.29 ± 0.35	1.64 ± 0.56
10	1.23 ± 0.16	1.54 ± 0.17
14	0.98 ± 0.09	1.21 ± 0.20
18	0.99 ± 0.12	1.19 ± 0.13
22	1.03 ± 0.14	1.30 ± 0.05
26	0.99 ± 0.34	1.15 ± 0.41
30	0.95 ± 0.20	0.82 ± 0.13
34	0.76 ± 0.10	0.43 ± 0.26
Overall	1.02 ± 0.24	1.17 ± 0.42

3 Constitutive Modeling of Degradation-Induced Changes in Scaffold Mechanics

The tensile test data were handled in Scilab (The Scilab Consortium, Domaine de Voluceau, France). Force values were filtered with a seven element triangular window moving average filter in order to remove test associated noise. Test sample dimensions and force-displacement data of strain $\varepsilon = 0$ to 20 % of the final extension were extracted from the Instron data files. From this force-displacement dataset, each sample was represented during characterisation by 11 points at equal spacing.

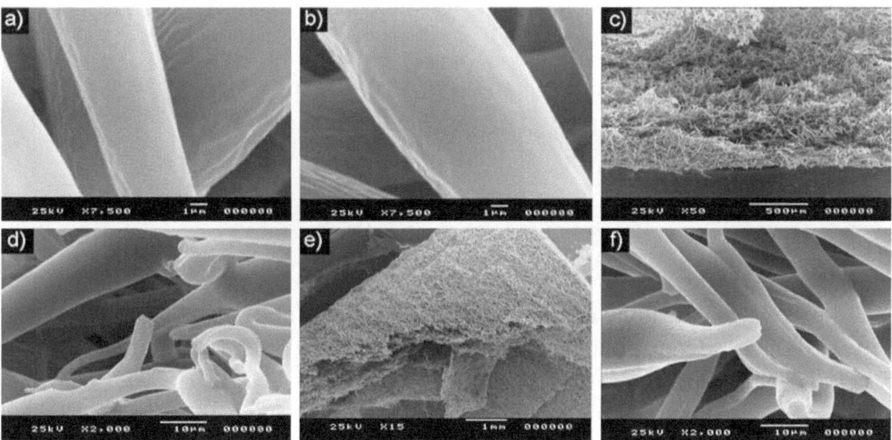

Fig. 8 SEM micrographs of electro-spun scaffold samples showing section of fibres after 14 days (a) and 34 days (b) of degradation before mechanical testing, and after degradation for 5 days (c, d) and 26 days (e, f) and subsequent mechanical testing to failure (The magnification and scale bar length are: **a**: ×7500, 1 µm; **b**: ×7500, 1 µm; **c**: ×50, 500 µm; **d**: ×2000, 10 µm; **e**: ×15, 1 mm; **f**: ×2000, 10 µm)

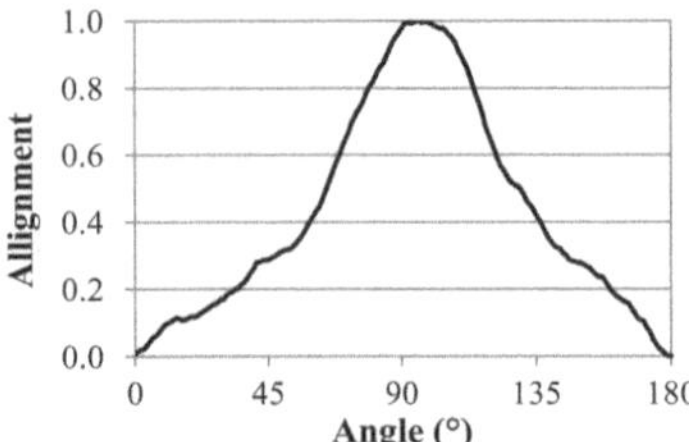

Fig. 9 Normalised amount of fibre alignment versus analysis angle for an electro-spun scaffold (outside surface) of Riboldi et al. determined with 2D FFT analysis of a published SEM micrograph, Fig. 1a in [12]. The analysis angles of 0° and 180° coincide with the longitudinal axis of the target mandrel, and electro-spun tube, whereas the angle of 90° refers to the circumferential direction. The distinguishing characteristic between the alignment distribution of Riboldi et al. compared to the current study was an increased concentration of alignment in spinning direction (90°) and absence of alignment in perpendicular direction (0°, 180°)

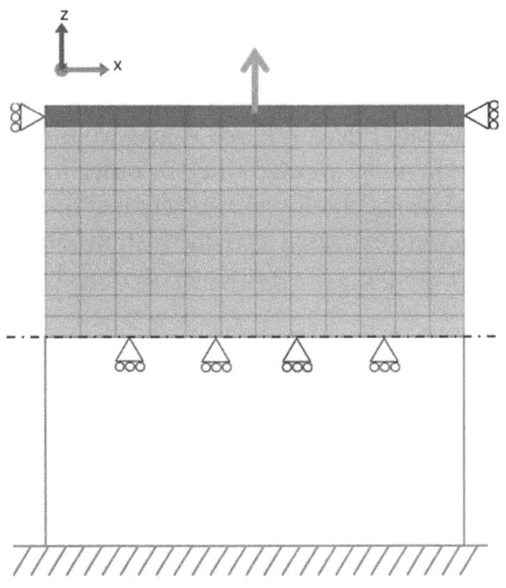

Fig. 10 Undeformed FE model representing one half of the axisymmetric geometry of the scaffold sample for uni-axial tensile testing

A uni-axial tensile finite element model in FEBio (University of Utah, Salt Lake City, USA) was used to simulate the mechanical tests in order to model the scaffold material. The model represented the scaffold with a $12 \times 5 \times 10$ ($x \times y \times z$) hexahedral element mesh with half-symmetry through the x–y plane illustrated in Fig. 10. Uni-axial loading was simulated by controlling the z-displacement of a rigid body tied to the top edge of the sample. For each physically tested sample, the mesh was resized and the deflection scaled based on the physical experiment.

A single-order, isotropic Ogden material was used, defined by the hyperelastic strain energy function:

$$W(\tilde{\lambda}_1, \tilde{\lambda}_2, \tilde{\lambda}_3) = \sum_{i=1}^{n} \frac{c_i}{m_i^2} \left(\tilde{\lambda}_1^{m_i} + \tilde{\lambda}_2^{m_i} + \tilde{\lambda}_3^{m_i} - 3 \right) + U(J) \tag{1}$$

where c_i and m_i are material coefficients, n is the order with $n = 1$, $\tilde{\lambda}_1$, $\tilde{\lambda}_2$ and $\tilde{\lambda}_3$ are the eigenvalues of the deviatoric right Cauchy deformation tensor, $U(J)$ is the volumetric component and J is the determinant of the deformation gradient.

Characterisation was performed on a per sample basis by fitting the mesh to the respective sample dimensions and loading the specific sample force-displacement data. The built-in functionality in FEBio was used to identify the constitutive coefficients c_i and m_i for an optimal match of numerical and experimental force-displacement data by minimising the objective function

$$\chi(\mathbf{a}) = \sum_{i=1}^{N} [\alpha_i]^2 \tag{2}$$

with

$$\alpha_i = y_i - y(x_i; \mathbf{a}) \tag{3}$$

where $y(x_i; \mathbf{a})$ is the function that describes the model, in this case the force-displacement data obtained from the FEM model, $\mathbf{a}$ is a vector with the unknown material properties (c_i and m_i), N is the number of data points, with $N = 11$ and (x_i, y_i) are the experimentally determined data.

Sample optimisation was run with a Scilab batch script. Two of the 45 samples were removed from the set due to invalid test data (one at $T = 18$ days) and sample failure prior to the final extension cycle (one at $T = 34$ days). Data from each degradation time point were grouped together and processed chronologically according to degradation time. The averaged values of c_i and m_i for one time period were used as the initial condition for the following batch of samples. The material properties and optimisation objective function results were recorded for each sample.

The accuracy of the material model was assessed by converting the objective function results into an approximated average force difference ΔF between the experimental and computed results

$$\Delta F \approx \sqrt{\frac{\chi}{N}}. \tag{4}$$

Using the cross-sectional area A of the sample, this force difference was converted to a stress difference $\Delta \sigma$ with

$$\Delta \sigma \approx \frac{\Delta F}{A}, \tag{5}$$

and subsequently normalised with respect to the maximum experimental stress in the sample

$$\psi = \frac{\Delta \sigma}{\sigma_{\mathrm{max.\,exp}}}. \tag{6}$$

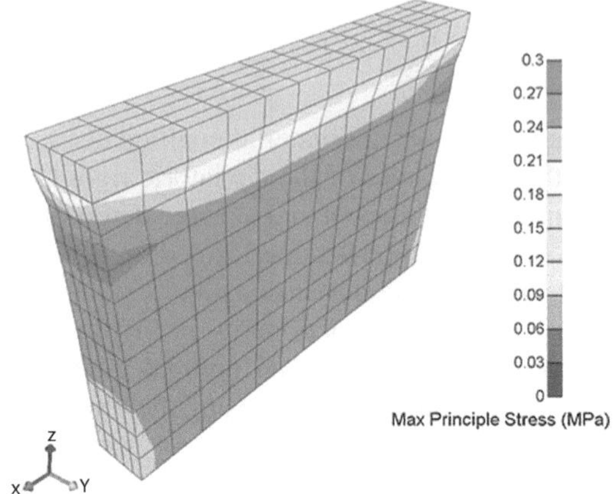

Fig. 11 Contour plot of maximum principal stress in the deformed uni-axial tensile test FE model

Table 2 Constitutive model parameters, experimental stress and normalised stress difference as measure for the model accuracy for non-degraded scaffold samples ($T = 0$) and after various periods of degradation (data are provided as mean $\pm$ stdev)

T (days)	Material coefficient c_1	Material coefficient m_1	Stress at 20 % strain $\sigma_{20\,\%,\mathrm{exp}}$ (kPa)	Normalised stress difference ψ (%)
0	0.167 ± 0.057	16.0 ± 2.6	136 ± 27	3.3 ± 0.6
5	0.331 ± 0.154	12.7 ± 2.2	196 ± 59	2.5 ± 0.7
10	0.236 ± 0.105	15.2 ± 3.4	180 ± 23	2.5 ± 0.6
14	0.146 ± 0.076	17.5 ± 5.2	137 ± 18	2.2 ± 0.6
18	0.208 ± 0.065	14.4 ± 2.0	150 ± 14	2.5 ± 0.6
22	0.103 ± 0.023	18.4 ± 1.4	123 ± 7.0	2.4 ± 0.7
26	0.157 ± 0.113	16.0 ± 2.3	129 ± 60	2.2 ± 0.5
30	0.040 ± 0.014	21.7 ± 3.1	72.0 ± 9.0	2.2 ± 0.5
34	0.008 ± 0.003	24.8 ± 7.6	29.0 ± 18	3.2 ± 2.3

Figure 11 illustrates the distribution of the maximum principle stress predicted in a sample utilising the optimised constitutive parameters. The optimisation successfully identified the constitutive coefficients c_1 and m_1 of the Ogden material model, for each of the degradation time points, to represent the non-linear force-displacement relationship of the scaffold with stiffening in the cyclic strain range observed in the experiments. The values for c_1 varied between 0.008 ± 0.003 and 0.331 ± 0.154, with a general trend of decreasing value with increasing degradation time (see Table 2). The values for m_1 ranged between 12.7 ± 2.2 and 24.8 ± 7.6, without exhibiting an apparent trend. The normalised difference between experimental and computed stress, ψ, used as indicator for the fitness of the model was found to be between 2.2 ± 0.5 % and 3.3 ± 0.6 % and is summarised in Table 2.

4 Discussion

The mechanical properties of the electro-spun DegraPol® scaffold deteriorated dramatically during the degradation period of 34 days. The maximum stress, σ_{max}, did not change significantly during the first 14 days of degradation but decreased steadily thereafter, dropping to 6.4 % of the initial value after 34 days. The strain, ε_{max}, associated with the maximum stress displayed a different change: from the start of the degradation it decreased rapidly to 26.4 % during the first 14 days and decreased markedly slower thereafter to 13.9 % after 34 days. The change in the strain ε_{max} coincided with the specification of the manufacturer that indicates complete degradation of DegraPol® DP30 with respect to the mechanical properties within two weeks. With increasing degradation time, the electro-spun scaffold became more susceptible to load cycling. A reduction of the stress at a strain of 20 % with repeated loading was observed in all samples. For degradation times of up to 18 days, the stress reduction was non-significant and resembled a mechanical conditioning which is also observed in other materials such as Nitinol [32] and biological soft tissues [33]. For a degradation time of 22 days and longer, the stress reduction became statistically significant, now governed by the reduced strength of the material. The elastic modulus also decreased with degradation time, the change was however less pronounced as that of the maximum stress and associated strain. The increase of the elastic modulus with increasing strain observed during the sixth loading cycle is typical feature of non-linear stiffening. Such a mechanical behaviour is observed in biological soft tissues such as arteries [34] and may be desirable for implant materials, e.g. biomedical coarse knit fabrics [16, 35], that aim at simulating physiological mechanics. The deterioration of physical properties due to degradation was not reflected in scaffold mass. The mass of the samples remained nearly constant over the entire degradation period.

In order to assess the data of mechanical characteristics of the current study against those reported in literature, scaffold structure and materials used need to be compared. The fibre thickness of the scaffold was found to be similar to electro-spun DegraPol® scaffolds used in previous studies [12, 20]. While the amount of fibre alignment appeared to be similar to that of the scaffold by Riboldi et al. [12] from visual inspection of SEM images, the 2D FFT analysis indicated a lower amount of alignment in the direction of rotation in the scaffold used in the current study. It was also found that the fibre alignment was more pronounced on the outer surface than on the inner surface. This can be explained with an increase in tangential velocity on the target surface during the spinning process that is associated with the increase in target diameter due to scaffold build-up, and which has been reported to affect fibre alignment [31].

The mechanical properties obtained for the non-degraded scaffold were lower compared to electro-spun DegraPol® DP15 [12]. The maximum stress, associated strain and elastic modulus reported were 4.8-, 1.25- and 6.26-fold ($\sigma_{max} = 2.52 \pm 0.17$ MPa, $\varepsilon_{max} = 220.40 \pm 57.09$ %, E $= 10.15 \pm 0.69$ MPa) of the values obtained in the current study. Since the ratio of hard- and soft segment of the two DegraPol® variants was identical (personal communications: S. Mantero, Politecnico di Milano, 23/06/2010; E. Bonavoglia, ab medica S.p.A, 28/06/2010), the higher mechanical properties of the scaffold of Riboldi et al. [12] were ascribed to a more pronounced fibre alignment (Fig. 9) [11, 31]. The apparent but non-significant improvements in mechanical property parameters σ_{max} and $\sigma_{20\,\%,i}$ after five days of degradation compared to the non-degraded scaffold (see Fig. 6(a) and (b), respectively) could be a result of the hydration of the samples. Non-degraded samples were not pre-wet prior to testing, and as the swelling of fibres during submersion could affect the mesh structure irreversibly [27].

The elastic modulus of electro-spun DegraPol® has previously been reported as being constant up to 10 % strain [12]. Although a constant elastic modulus—be it in bulk or processed form of the material—gives an indication of the material stiffness [12, 19, 20], more in depth information is beneficial for constitutive modelling and computational mechanics. The analysis carried out in the current study indicated a variation of the elastic modulus both with the change in magnitude of strain and the number of loadings. For the initial loading, the elastic modulus was found to increase on average by 91 % with the strain increasing from 0 % to 8 % while it decreased from this maximum value by 27 % with the strain further increasing to 18 %. A different characteristic was observed during the final loading with the elastic modulus steadily increasing by 501 % with the strain increasing from 0 % to 18 %. This pattern was found for the non-degraded scaffold as well as for all degradation time points. Similar changes of the elastic modulus with strain and effects of load cycling were reported for electro-spun polycaprolactone (PCL) for a strain up to 35 % [22].

The lack of mass loss indicated that the degradation occurred on a molecular level only but did not progress far enough to cause a significant volume of fibres to dissolve or break off. This is supported by the SEM micrographs which did not show significant fibre surface changes between samples after 34 days degradation and non-degraded samples. Lendlein et al. [19] and Riboldi et al. [12] reported a reduction in molecular mass immediately after the start of the degradation. However, a reduction in sample mass has been reported to commence only between 28 and more than 100 days after degradation onset depending on the specific DegraPol® version tested [19]. The reduction in molecular mass without loss in scaffold mass in the early stages of degradation has been reported to be caused by random hydrolytic cleavage of the macromolecular chains. The loss of sample mass commenced once the molecular mass dropped below a certain threshold at which polymer segments became small enough to filter out of the bulk polymer [19]. Furthermore, significant changes in mechanical strength were reported in the same time period as molecular mass changes [12, 19, 27]. This indicates that a change in mass, or lack thereof, of a sample is not an appropriate measure of the degree of degradation with respect to mechanical properties. It is however important to investigate the loss in sample mass, and material volume, as an indication of space available for ingrowth of cells and tissue.

During tensile testing of the scaffolds after longer degradation times, it was found that some samples exhibited severe plastic deformation (see Fig. 8(d, f)), disintegration and, in some instances, failure during one of the load cycles, i.e. prior to the final loading. For future studies, a decrease of the upper strain limit of $\varepsilon = 20\,\%$ for the load cycles may be considered to prevent excessive plastic deformation during cycling and to determine the change of the elastic limit of the scaffold with progressing degradation. When evaluating the increasing lack of structural stability of the degrading scaffold, the potential mechanical effect of tissue regenerating in the scaffold needs to be considered. For the design of a tissue regenerating implant, the structural degradation of the scaffold needs to be adjusted to the rate of tissue regeneration so as to prevent structural failure of the implant. If this is not feasible, alternative designs need to ensure structural integrity of the implant, for example composite structures comprising two or more components.

The normalised stress difference ψ indicated a good model accuracy and successful representation of the constitutive scaffold properties including the effects of degradation. The material coefficient c_1 followed the same trend with degradation time as the tensile stress at 20 % strain, $\sigma_{20\ \%,\mathrm{exp}}$, with an overall decrease of c_1 and stress with increasing degradation time (see Table 2). This observation was, however, not true on a time-point to time-point basis. The latter was ascribed to inconsistencies possibly in the manufacture and testing procedures that need addressing in future work.

This study was a first step to extend the research in mechanics and constitutive modelling of degrading tissue regenerative scaffolds. Future studies with extensions of the work presented, e.g. use of physiological degradation solution such as phosphate buffered saline, characterisation of molecular weight of the scaffold, and changes thereof during degradation, will provide important additional data. With the aim of developing more comprehensive constitutive models for scaffold-based soft tissue regeneration, further research will also address important aspects such as strain rate sensitivity of the scaffold material, effect of tissue incorporation and application-specific mechanics.

Acknowledgements The authors thank ab medica S.p.A for donating the DegraPol® material for this study. ETH Zurich and University of Zurich are owners and ab medica S.p.A is exclusive licensee of all IP Rights of DegraPol®.

Funding Sources This study was supported financially by the National Research Foundation (NRF) of South Africa. Any opinion, findings and conclusions or recommendations expressed in this publication are those of the authors and therefore the NRF does not accept any liability in regard thereto. HK received a Matching Dissertation Grant from the International Society of Biomechanics.

References

1. Furth ME, Atala A, Van Dyke ME (2007) Smart biomaterials design for tissue engineering and regenerative medicine. Biomaterials 28(34):5068–5073
2. Williams DF (2006) To engineer is to create: the link between engineering and regeneration. Trends Biotechnol 24(1):4–8
3. Zilla P, Bezuidenhout D, Human P (2007) Prosthetic vascular grafts: wrong models, wrong questions and no healing. Biomaterials 28(34):5009–5027

4. Bezuidenhout D, Davies N, Zilla P (2002) Effect of well defined dodecahedral porosity on inflammation and angiogenesis. ASAIO J 48(5):465–471
5. Davies N, Dobner S, Bezuidenhout D, Schmidt C, Beck M, Zisch AH et al (2008) The dosage dependence of VEGF stimulation on scaffold neovascularisation. Biomaterials 29(26):3531–3538
6. Hou Q, Grijpma DW, Feijen J (2003) Porous polymeric structures for tissue engineering prepared by a coagulation, compression moulding and salt leaching technique. Biomaterials 24(11):1937–1947
7. Yoon JJ, Park TG (2001) Degradation behaviors of biodegradable macroporous scaffolds prepared by gas foaming of effervescent salts. J Biomed Mater Res 55(3):401–408
8. Sarkar S, Burriesci G, Wojcik A, Aresti N, Hamilton G, Seifalian AM (2009) Manufacture of small calibre quadruple lamina vascular bypass grafts using a novel automated extrusion-phase-inversion method and nanocomposite polymer. J Biomech 42(6):722–730
9. Guan J, Fujimoto KL, Sacks MS, Wagner WR (2005) Preparation and characterization of highly porous, biodegradable polyurethane scaffolds for soft tissue applications. Biomaterials 26(18):3961–3971
10. McClure MJ, Sell SA, Simpson DG, Walpoth BH, Bowlin GL (2010) A three-layered electrospun matrix to mimic native arterial architecture using polycaprolactone, elastin, and collagen: a preliminary study. Acta Biomater 6(7):2422–2433
11. Ayres CE, Bowlin GL, Henderson SC, Taylor L, Shultz J, Alexander J, Telemeco TA, Simpson DG (2006) Modulation of anisotropy in electrospun tissue-engineering scaffolds: analysis of fiber alignment by the fast Fourier transform. Biomaterials 27(32):5524–5534
12. Riboldi SA, Sampaolesi M, Neuenschwander P, Cossu G, Mantero S (2005) Electrospun degradable polyesterurethane membranes: potential scaffolds for skeletal muscle tissue engineering. Biomaterials 26(22):4606–4615
13. Holzapfel GA, Gasser TC, Ogden RW (2000) A new constitutive framework for arterial wall mechanics and a comparative study of material models. J Elast 61(1–3):1–48
14. Shadwick RE (1999) Mechanical design in arteries. J Exp Biol 202(Pt 23):3305–3313
15. Steinman DA, Vorp DA, Ethier CR (2003) Computational modeling of arterial biomechanics: insights into pathogenesis and treatment of vascular disease. J Vasc Surg 37(5):1118–1128
16. Yeoman MS, Reddy BD, Bowles H, Zilla P, Bezuidenhout D, Franz T (2009) The use of finite element methods and genetic algorithms in search of an optimal fabric reinforced porous graft system. Ann Biomed Eng 37(11):2266–2287
17. Zidi M, Cheref M (2003) Mechanical analysis of a prototype of small diameter vascular prosthesis: Numerical simulations. Comput Biol Med 33(1):65–75
18. Di Prima M, Gall K, McDowell DL, Guldberg R, Lin A, Sanderson T, Campbell D, Arzberger SC (2010) Deformation of epoxy shape memory polymer foam. Part I: Experiments and macroscale constitutive modeling. Mech Mater 42(3):304–314
19. Lendlein A, Colussi M, Neuenschwander P, Suter UW (2001) Hydrolytic degradation of phase-segregated multiblock copoly(ester urethane)s containing weak links. Macromol Chem Phys 202(13):2702–2711
20. Lendlein A, Neuenschwander P, Suter UW (1998) Tissue-compatible multiblock copolymers for medical applications, controllable in degradation rate and mechanical properties. Macromol Chem Phys 199(12):2785–2796
21. Kwon IK, Kidoaki S, Matsuda T (2005) Electrospun nano- to microfiber fabrics made of biodegradable copolyesters: structural characteristics, mechanical properties and cell adhesion potential. Biomaterials 26(18):3929–3939
22. Duling RR, Dupaix RB, Katsube N, Lannutti J (2008) Mechanical characterization of electrospun polycaprolactone (PCL): a potential scaffold for tissue engineering. J Biomech Eng 130(1):011006 (13 pp)
23. Lee SJ, Liu J, Oh SH, Soker S, Atala A, Yoo JJ (2008) Development of a composite vascular scaffolding system that withstands physiological vascular conditions. Biomaterials 29(19):2891–2898

24. Vaz CM, van Tuijl S, Bouten CVC, Baaijens FPT (2005) Design of scaffolds for blood vessel tissue engineering using a multi-layering electrospinning technique. Acta Biomater 1(5):575–582
25. Mirensky TL, Fein CW, Nguyen GK, Hibino N, Sawh-Martinez RF, Yi T, McGillicuddy EA, Villalona G, Shinoka T, Breuer CK (2009) Characterization of small-diameter electrospun tissue-engineered arterial grafts. J Am Coll Surg 209(3):S30
26. Kang Y, Yao Y, Yin G, Huang Z, Liao X, Xu X, Zhao G (2009) A study on the in vitro degradation properties of poly(l-lactic acid)/[beta]-tricalcium phosphate(PLLA/[beta]-TCP) scaffold under dynamic loading. Med Eng Phys 31(5):589–594
27. Henry JA, Simonet M, Pandit A, Neuenschwander P (2007) Characterization of a slowly degrading biodegradable polyesterurethane for tissue engineering scaffolds. J Biomed Mater Res, Part A 82A(3):669–679
28. Bonchek LI (1980) Prevention of endothelial damage during preparation of saphenous veins for bypass grafting. J Thorac Cardiovasc Surg 79(6):911–915
29. Milleret V, Simonet M, Bittermann AG, Neuenschwander P, Hall H (2009) Cyto- and hemocompatibility of a biodegradable 3d-scaffold material designed for medical applications. J Biomed Mater Res, Part B, Appl Biomater 91(1):109–121
30. Ayres CE, Jha BS, Meredith H, Bowman JR, Bowlin GL, Henderson SC, Simpson DG (2008) Measuring fiber alignment in electrospun scaffolds: a user's guide to the 2d fast Fourier transform approach. J Biomater Sci Polymer Ed 19(5):603–621
31. Ayres CE, Bowlin GL, Pizinger R, Taylor LT, Keen CA, Simpson DG (2007) Incremental changes in anisotropy induce incremental changes in the material properties of electrospun scaffolds. Acta Biomater 3(5):651–661
32. van der Merwe H, Reddy BD, Zilla P, Bezuidenhout D, Franz T (2008) A computational study of knitted nitinol meshes for their prospective use as external vein reinforcement. J Biomech 41(6):1302–1309
33. Carew EO, Barber JE, Vesely I (2000) Role of preconditioning and recovery time in repeated testing of aortic valve tissues: validation through quasilinear viscoelastic theory. Ann Biomed Eng 28(9):1093–1100
34. Valdez-Jasso D, Bia D, Zócalo Y, Armentano R, Haider M, Olufsen M (2011) Linear and nonlinear viscoelastic modeling of aorta and carotid pressure–area dynamics under *in vivo* and *ex vivo* conditions. Ann Biomed Eng 39(5):1438–1456
35. Yeoman MS, Reddy D, Bowles HC, Bezuidenhout D, Zilla P, Franz T (2010) A constitutive model for the warp-weft coupled non-linear behavior of knitted biomedical textiles. Biomaterials 31(32):8484–8493

4D Numerical Analysis of Scaffolds:
A New Approach

A.C. Vieira, A.T. Marques, R.M. Guedes, and V. Tita

Abstract A large range of biodegradable polymers are used to produce scaffolds for tissue engineering, which temporarily replace the biomechanical functions of a biologic tissue while it progressively regenerates its capacities. However, the mechanical behavior of biodegradable materials during its degradation, which is an important aspect of the scaffold design, is still an unexplored subject. For a biodegradable scaffold, performance will decrease along its degradation, ideally in accordance to the regeneration of the biologic tissue, avoiding the stress shielding effect or the premature rupture. In this chapter, a new numerical approach to predict the mechanical behavior of complex 3D scaffolds during degradation time (the 4th dimension) is presented. The degradation of mechanical properties should ideally be compatible to the tissue regeneration. With this new approach, an iterative process of optimization is possible to achieve an ideal solution in terms of mechanical behavior and degradation time. The scaffold can therefore be pre-validated in terms of functional compatibility. An example of application of this approach is demonstrated at the end of this chapter.

1 Introduction

There are many biodegradable polymers commercially available to produce a wide variety of scaffolds, each of them with suitable properties, according to the tissue they are supporting during regeneration. Many examples can be found from generic

A.C. Vieira (✉)
UMEC, Institute of Mechanical Engineering and Industrial Management, Rua Dr. Roberto Frias 378, 4200-465 Porto, Portugal
e-mail: avieira@inegi.up.pt

A.C. Vieira · A.T. Marques · R.M. Guedes
DEMec, Mechanical Engineering Department, Faculty of Engineering of the University of Porto (FEUP), University of Porto, Rua Dr. Roberto Frias, 4200-465, Porto, Portugal

V. Tita
Aeronautical Engineering Department, Engineering School of São Carlos, University of São Paulo, Av. Trabalhador São-carlense, 400, 13566-590, São Carlos, SP, Brazil

P.R. Fernandes, P.J. Bártolo (eds.), *Tissue Engineering*,
Computational Methods in Applied Sciences 31, DOI 10.1007/978-94-007-7073-7_4,
© Springer Science+Business Media Dordrecht 2014

tissue engineering scaffolds [24], biodegradable ligaments [51], biodegradable endovascular [8] and urethral stents [42]. The design process must contemplate the biocompatibility issues related to toxicity and the functional aspect related to mechanical considerations. In terms of mechanical dimensioning, one must consider not only the static strength and stiffness of the device, but also the long-term mechanical behavior considering degradation. This degradation is defined as the time-dependent cumulative irreversible damage due to hydrolysis.

When loading conditions are simple and the desired time for mechanical support is known, a "trial and error" approach may be enough to design reasonable reliable scaffolds. In more complex situations, engineers and designers can use numerical approaches to define the material formulation and geometry that will satisfy the immediate needs of symptomatic relief, without the occurrence of any degradation, using conventional dimensioning. However, the lack of design tools to predict long term behavior has limited the success of biodegradable scaffolds. The considerations and the dimensioning methods developed until this moment may overcome this limitation, normally, providing a poor solution. Therefore, it is necessary to propose new approaches to improve the solution for this problem.

In this chapter, a new numerical approach, which can use hyper elastic constitutive models, such as the Neo-Hookean, the Mooney-Rivlin and the second reduced order will be discussed. In fact, the new approach consists on a constitutive model and a failure criterion, which are implemented in commercial finite element software packages like ABAQUS via User Material (UMAT) subroutine and Python language. Through a failure criterion, the degradation rate was used to define the strength of the material at a given degradation time, using a first order kinetic equation. The material parameters of the constitutive model were calculated by inverse parameterization of the model compared against experimental data. It was found that only one material parameter varies linearly with the hydrolytic damage (which depends on the degradation time). Although this approach was evaluated based on experimental tensile tests of fibers, for a particular blend of polylactic acid (PLA) and polycaprolactone (PCL), the authors believe that this can be extended to other thermoplastic biodegradable materials with response similar to hyper elastic behavior. The new numerical approach was able to predict the load-displacement plot with reasonable accuracy until 50 % of hydrolytic damage. It can be further extended to numerical 3D models and complex loading scenarios for different applications, to predict the long-term mechanical behavior.

2 Biodegradable Polymers

Biodegradable polymers can be classified as either naturally derived polymers or synthetic polymers. A large range of mechanical properties and degradation rates are possible among these polymers. However, each of these may have some shortcomings, which restrict its use for a specific application, due to inappropriate stiffness or degradation rate. Blending, copolymerization or composite techniques are extremely promising strategies, which can be used to tune the original mechanical and degradation properties of the polymers [1] according to the application requirements. The most popular and important class of biodegradable synthetic polymers are aliphatic polyesters, such as polylactic acid (PLLA and PDLA), polyglycolic acid (PGA), polycaprolactone (PCL), polyhydroxyalkanoates (PHA's) and polyethylene oxide (PEO) among others. They can be processed like other thermoplastic materials.

The poly-α-hydroxyesters, PLA, PGA and their copolymers are the most popular aliphatic polyesters that have been synthesized for more than 30 years. The left-handed (L-lactide) and right-handed (D-lactide) are the two enantiomeric forms of PLA, with PDLA having a much higher degradation rate than PLLA, but similar initial mechanical properties. An exhaustive overview was done by Auras et al. [2]. PLLA is a rather brittle polymer with a low degradation rate, and compounding with PCL is frequently employed to improve mechanical properties. PCL is also hydrophobic with a low degradation rate, much more ductile than PLA [40]. PGA, since it is a hydrophilic material presents a high degradation rate. It is stiffer than PLA. The combination of PGA with PLA is usually employed to tune degradation rate [32]. Polyhydoxyalkanoates (PHA's) is the largest class of aliphatic polyesters, comprising poly 3-hydroxybutyrate (PHB), copolymers of 3-hydroxybutyrate and 3-hydroxyvalerate (PHBV), poly 4-hydroxybutyrate (P4HB), copolymers of 3-hydroxybutyrate and 3-hydroxyhexanoate (PHBHHx) and poly 3-hydroxyoctanoate (PHO) and its blends. The changing PHA compositions also allow favorable mechanical properties and degradation times within desirable time frames [6]. Natural polymers used in scaffolds include starch, collagen, silk, alginate, agarose, chitosan, fibrin, cellulosic, hyaluronic acid-based materials, among others. Some of these are bioactive materials, and their degradation products can modulate the inflammatory response. However, these are more prone to enzymatic degradation than the synthetic biodegradable polymers, consequently the degradation kinetics depends more on the host. The synthetic polymers have that advantage of more predictable behavior evolution. New biodegradable material solutions are continuously arising each day.

Presently 3D scaffolds can be printed with layers and parts of different biodegradable materials. These can then be coated with a biodegradable and bioactive material, to obtain a more intelligent surface in terms of cell mediated interaction. A complex geometry like these can be modeled in a commercial 3D drawing software and the mechanical behavior can be predicted by numerical simulation.

3 Biodegradation and Erosion

All biodegradable polymers contain hydrolysable or oxydable bonds. This makes the material sensitive to moisture, heat, light and also mechanical stresses. These different types of polymer degradation mechanisms (photo, thermal, mechanical and chemical degradation) can be present alone or combined, working synergistically to

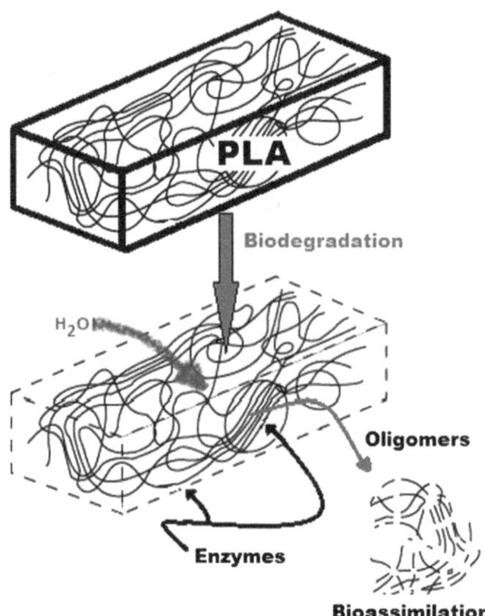

Fig. 1 Scheme of erosion process

the degradation. Usually, the most important degradation mechanism of biodegradable polymers is chemical degradation via hydrolysis or enzyme-catalyzed hydrolysis [14]. The most important factor is its chemical structure and the occurrence of specific bonds along its chains. Like those in groups of esters, amides, etc., which might be susceptible to hydrolysis when exposed to water [18, 33].

Another important distinction must be made between erosion and degradation. Both are irreversible processes. However, while the degree of erosion is estimated from the mass loss, the degree of degradation can be estimated by measuring the evolution of molecular weight, by SEC (Size Exclusion Chromatography) or GPC (Gel Permeation Chromatography), or the tensile strength evolution (by universal tensile testing). Hence, the hydrolytic degradation process is included on the erosion process.

The erosion process can be described by phenomenological diffusion-reaction mechanisms presented in Fig. 1. An aqueous media diffuses into the polymeric material while oligomeric products diffuse outwards to be then bio-assimilated by the host environment. Then, there is material erosion with correspondent mass loss. On the other hand, degradation refers to mechanical damage and depends on hydrolysis. Within the polymeric matrix, hydrolytic reactions take place, mediated by water and/or enzymes. While water diffuses rapidly well inside the material, enzymes are large molecules unable to do it, and so they degrade at surface. The degradation of polyesters by micro-organisms is initiated by extracellular hydrolases, which are secreted by the organisms to reduce the molar mass of the polymeric substrate and to make it bio-available and bio-assimilated. It was demonstrated by Tokiwa and Suzuki [44] that synthetic polyesters can be attacked by hydrolases (lipases). However, for most biodegradable materials, especially synthetic polymers, passive hydrolysis due to the presence of water molecules is the most important mode of degradation.

To fully model the erosion process, a complex mathematical model is needed to account for all the reaction steps and for the structural and morphologic details. The parameters in such a model require extensive experimentation. Numerical techniques have been used [5, 15, 17, 29, 56, 58] to solve the corresponding equations for devices of both simple and complicated geometries, in the context of drug release systems. However, these models did not account for the mechanical properties degradation of these devices.

Polymer degradation is the first step of the erosion phenomenon. The complete erosion of the polymer is known to take substantially longer than the complete loss of tensile strength. During this first phase, aqueous solution penetrates the polymer, followed by hydrolytic degradation, converting these very long polymer chains into shorter water-soluble fragments, which can be regarded as a reverse polycondensation process. For example, PLA becomes soluble in water for molecular weight, M_n, below ≈ 20.000 (g/mol) [59].

4 Hydrolytic Damage

Hydrolytic damage can be defined as the time-dependent cumulative irreversible damage due to the hydrolytic cleavage of polymeric molecules. After immersion of a biodegradable polymeric device in an aqueous medium, water uptake is the very first event that occurs, up to a saturation of water concentration that depends on the hydrophilicity of the polymer, its crystalline degree, the temperature, pH and flow of the media. This step is accompanied by volume expansion due to the fluid ingress, usually designated by swelling. The intrusion of water then triggers the chemical polymer degradation, leading to the scission of molecules and the creation of oligomers. The penetrating water rapidly creates a negative gradient of water concentrations from the surface to the centre as expected from a pure diffusion viewpoint. However, this gradient vanishes in a couple of hours or days, when the specimen saturates. Diffusion of small molecules like water is rather fast as compared with degradation that can take several months. Therefore, one can consider that hydrolysis of ester bonds starts homogeneously along the volume from the beginning, promoting bulk erosion [25]. This assumption is very precise for small thickness devices, such as fibers or films. Water uptake can also lead to further recrystallization of the polymer. Water acts as a plasticizer, lowering the glass transition temperature and softening the material.

The water concentration (w) along the thickness, and during incubation, is determined using Fick's equation:

$$\frac{dw}{dt} = D_1 \frac{\partial^2 w}{\partial x^2} + D_2 \frac{\partial^2 w}{\partial y^2} + D_3 \frac{\partial^2 w}{\partial z^2} \tag{1}$$

In the case of isotropic polymers, diffusion has no preferential direction, and $D_1 = D_2 = D_3 = D$. The diffusion coefficient D of the material can be determined

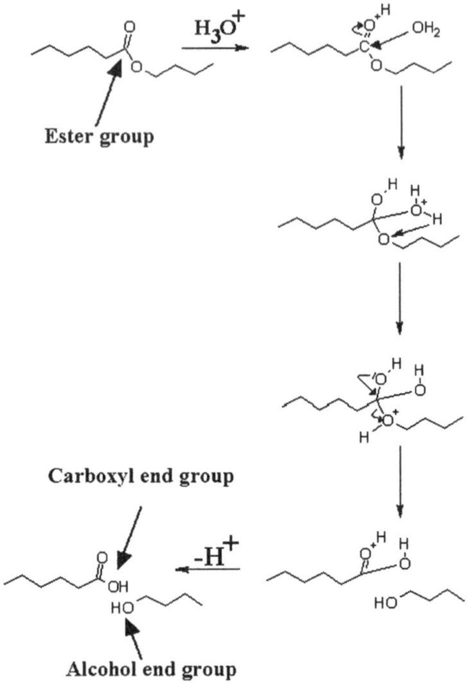

 A.C. Vieira et al.

Fig. 2 Acid catalyzed
hydrolysis mechanism [31]

by inverse parameterization, measuring the increase in weight due to moisture absorption during incubation, on samples with two different diameters. The amount of absorbed water is computed from:

$$m_w = 100 * (m_{ws} - m_{wr})/m_{wr} \tag{2}$$

where m_{wr} and m_{ws} are the weights of the specimen before and after absorption, respectively.

The macromolecular skeleton of many polymers comprises chemical bonds (e.g. polyethylene terephthalate PET, polybutylene terephthalate PBT, epoxies crosslinked by anhydrides, unsaturated polyesters, vinylesters, PLA, PGA, PCL and PHA's), such as ester groups, that can go through hydrolysis in the presence of water molecules, leading to chain scissions. In the case of polylactides, these scissions occur at the ester groups. Ester hydrolysis can be either acid or base catalyzed [41]. In Fig. 2, a scheme of the acid based hydrolysis mechanism, more common in PLA degradation, is presented. A general consequence of such a process is the lowering of the plastic flow ability of the polymer, thus causing the change of a ductile, tough behavior into a brittle one. If the behavior was initially brittle, there will be an increase in the brittleness. Each polymer molecule, with its own carboxylic and alcohol end groups, is broken in two, randomly in the middle at a given ester group. So, while the molecules are being splitted by hydrolysis the number of carboxylic end groups will increase with degradation time (see Fig. 2).

Hydrolysis has traditionally been modeled using a first order kinetics equation based on the kinetic mechanism of hydrolysis, according to the Michaelis–Menten scheme [4]. According to Farrar and Gilson [12], the following first-order equation describes the hydrolytic process relative to the carboxyl end groups (C), ester concentration (E) and water concentration (w):

$$\frac{dC}{dt} = kEwC = uC \tag{3}$$

where u is the hydrolysis rate of the material, k is the hydrolysis rate constant, assuming that E and w are constant in the early stages of the reaction. In addition, water is spread out uniformly in the sample volume (no diffusion control).

Or using the scission number n_t per mass unit, as presented in the literature [4], at time t is given, and the initial concentration of carboxyl end groups C_0 is known, Eq. (3) becomes:

$$\frac{dn_t}{dt} = kEw(C_0 + n_t) \tag{4}$$

The experimental measurement of molecular weights allows the determination of n_t, and consequently the degradation rate constant:

$$n_t = \frac{1}{M_{n_t}} - \frac{1}{M_{n_0}} \tag{5}$$

Using the molecular weight, and since the concentrations of carboxyl end groups are given by $C = 1/M_n$, Eq. (3) becomes:

$$M_{n_t} = M_{n_0} e^{-ut} \tag{6}$$

where M_{n_t} and M_{n_0}, are the number-average molecular weight, at a given time t and initially at $t = 0$, respectively. This equation leads to a relationship $M_n = f(t)$, and the result is in g/mol. However, in the design phase of a tissue engineering biodegradable device, it is important to predict the evolution of mechanical properties like tensile strength, instead of molecular weight. It has been shown [57] that the fracture strength of a generic thermoplastic polymer can, in many cases, be related to M_n through the empirical relationship:

$$\sigma = \sigma_\infty - \frac{A}{M_{n_t}} = \sigma_\infty - \frac{A}{M_{n_0} e^{-ut}} \tag{7}$$

where σ is the fracture strength, σ_∞ is the fracture strength at infinite molecular weight, and A is a material constant. Equation (7) provides a description of the time dependence of the material's mechanical strength, which is relevant in the design phase of a biodegradable device. Since this is an empirical equation, constant A must be determined experimentally for each material. One can thus determine the limit strength of the device during the recovering of the tissue, $\sigma_d = f(t)$. When regenerating a tissue, the strength of the scaffold, σ_d, should be compatible to the strength of the new formed tissue $\sigma_l = \sigma(t)$. According to Farrar and Gilson [12], the hydrolysis rate depends on the structure of the polymer, and is independent of its initial molecular weight. Equation (7) is illustrated in Fig. 3.

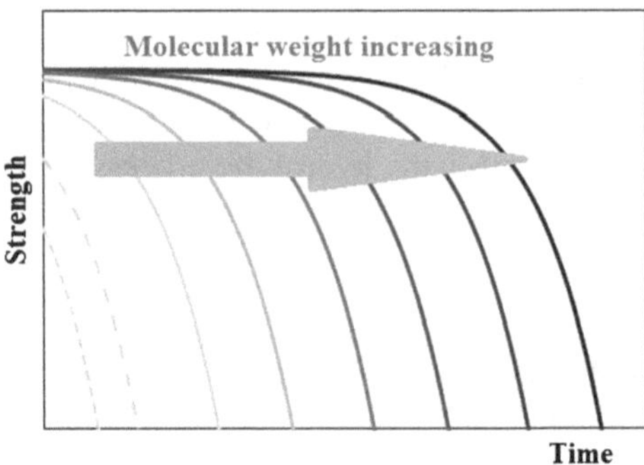

Fig. 3 Tensile strength vs. time for different initial molecular weight (based on [12])

The storage or sterilization processes may pre-degrade the material, leading to reduction of degradation time and its initial mechanical strength, but the rate of degradation remains the same. To tune degradation time, specimens with different initial molecular weight can be created by gamma-irradiation starting from commercial materials available. Regrettably, this technique also reduces the initial mechanical properties of the materials.

Equation (7) is not a very good model for tensile strength, except in the brittle failure regime for amorphous polymers or semi-crystalline polymers below their glass transition temperature. This is a common problem with highly ductile polymers. In these cases, it is more correct to use true values instead of nominal stress and strain, by assuming that the deformation occurs at constant volume [57]. In this case, the true area, A, is given by $A_0/(1+\varepsilon)$; where A_0 is the initial area and ε is the nominal strain. This leads to the true stress being given by $(1+\varepsilon)*\sigma_a$; where σ_a is the apparent stress based on A_0.

As it will be shown in the next sections, strength follows the same trend as the molecular weight:

$$\sigma_t = \sigma_0 * e^{-ut} \tag{8}$$

The hydrolytic damage, defined by the ratio between the initial strength of the virgin material and the current strength, after a certain degradation time, is:

$$d_h = 1 - \frac{\sigma_t}{\sigma_0} = 1 - e^{-ut} = 1 - e^{-kEwt} \tag{9}$$

So the hydrolytic damage depends on the hydrolysis kinetic constant, k, the concentrations of ester groups, E, the water concentration in the polymer matrix, w, and the degradation time t. The hydrolysis kinetic constant, k, is a thermodynamic quantity associated with the probability of molecular scission, and it depends on temperature, load applied to the material and pH of the aqueous media. The pH of the aqueous medium also affects the hydrolysis reaction rates [21]. Tsuji et al. studied the hydrolysis of PLLA films at 37 °C in alkaline solution (pH 12) [45], acid solution (pH 2.0) [47] and phosphate-buffered solutions (pH 7.4) [46]. In the human body, pH can be considered constant, kept by the organism at a homeostatic value.

Temperature will augment diffusion due to increased molecular flexibility, but it will also amplify the hydrolysis rate, due to excitement of the molecules that it will raise the probability of bond scissions. Also, in the human body, temperature is kept constant at the homeostatic value of around 37 °C. The influence of the mechanical environment in the hydrolysis rate was also reported [7, 30]. Loaded fibers degrade faster than unloaded ones, and the magnitude of degradation depends on the level of applied stress and the incubation time. Similarly to temperature, stress also increases the probability of bond scissions. In most applications, the material is submitted to a stress state. When the stress state remains constant during degradation, the hydrolysis rate must be determined for that particular load case. If any variation were to occur in the stress state, temperature, or environment, k would no longer be constant.

In this example, homogeneous degradation with instant diffusion, the hydrolysis rate, u, is constant, and damage only depends on degradation time. Although, these considerations are valid in the majority of the cases, in some cases, the hydrolysis rate cannot be considered constant. In brief, the hydrolysis rate of the material (u) should be determined experimentally in accordance to the degradation environment of the application. In the characterization section, an example degradation rate determination will be presented.

5 Further Refinements of Degradation Models

In a complex organism, several substances are responsible for degradation. More precise models can include each one of these substances. Bioprocess models are often restricted to the evolution of macroscopic species involved in a reaction scheme [3]. Such a reaction scheme describes the main phenomena occurring in the culture and is typically built of a reduced number of irreversible reactions involving macroscopic species. For each enzyme and water, its hydrolytic effect is usually modeled, using a first order differential equation, with different hydrolytic constant rates and concentrations that must be known. The model used is formally based on the kinetic mechanism of enzymatic hydrolysis according to the Michaelis–Menten scheme [48]:

$$Z + S \underset{k-1}{\overset{k1}{\rightleftharpoons}} ZS$$
$$ZS \overset{k2}{\longrightarrow} P + Z$$

(10)

where Z and S represent the enzyme and substrate polymer, respectively and ZS is the enzyme/substrate complex, P is used to denote the hydrolysis reaction products, $k1$, $k-1$ and $k2$ are rate parameters. $k1$ describes the diffusion and adsorption of the enzyme onto the substrate polymer, $k-1$ the dissociation of the ZS complex without degradation (in general, equal to zero) [48] and $k2$ the degradation process. The degradation is mostly assumed to be the rate-limiting step, because equilibrium in adsorption is much faster compared to degradation.

In order to perform computer simulation based on these models, the equations can be discretized using the mixed finite element method for the space and an implicit scheme for the time. Having determined the concentration of the carboxylic end groups at the nth discrete time point, the degradation equation can be solved and it can proceed to the next time step (or increment).

When a process is composed of a sequence of reactions, the overall rate is determined by the slowest reaction, named the rate-limiting step [19]. Klyosov and Rabinowitch [22] reported that the rate limiting step may change between the beginning of the reaction and after a certain degree of substrate conversion.

The degree of crystallinity may also be a crucial factor, since hydrolysis occurs mainly in the amorphous domains. Water and enzymes degrade the more accessible amorphous region, but are unable to attack the less accessible crystalline portions. The water permeability along the crystalline region is much smaller than amorphous region. The observed increase in percentage of the crystalline phase is explained by the faster degradation that occurs in the amorphous region. Polymers with low crystallinity showed increased hydrolysis rates [36, 37]. As the crystallinity increases steadily throughout the reaction, substrate becomes increasingly resistant to further hydrolysis [10, 11], therefore affecting the kinetics of the process [20, 55]. To model this phenomenon, knowing the initial crystalline degree, two different rates can be considered for both phases, and two different hydrolytic damage values should be calculated and added according to the volume fractions. The crystallinity of copolymers (X %) can be determined by dividing the observed heat of fusion in a DSC (Differential Scanning Calorimetry) test, by the theoretical value for perfectly crystalline polymer according to:

$$X \% = \frac{\Delta h_m}{\Delta h_m^0} \tag{11}$$

Crystallinity also affects the mechanical properties of materials. Their glass transition temperature is lowered due to water uptake, which can lead to recrystallization of the polymer. Hence, material processing and storage conditions have a great influence on mechanical and degradation properties [35].

6 Surface vs. Bulk Erosion

All degradable polymers share the property of eroding upon degradation. The water ingress triggers the chemical polymer degradation leading to the creation of oligomers and monomers. Progressive degradation changes the microstructure of the bulk through the formation of pore via which oligomers are released. Concomitantly, the pH inside pores begins to be controlled by degradation products, which typically have some acid-base functionality. Finally, oligomers and monomers are released, leading to the weight loss of polymer devices. The distinction made between surface (or heterogeneous) and bulk (or homogeneous) eroding materials is used to classify degradable polymers.

Different types of erosion are illustrated in Fig. 4. In Fig. 4c, there is a typical case of homogeneous or bulk erosion without autocatalysis, in which diffusion occurs instantaneously. Hence, the decrease in molecular weight, the reduction in mechanical properties, and the loss of mass occur simultaneously throughout the entire

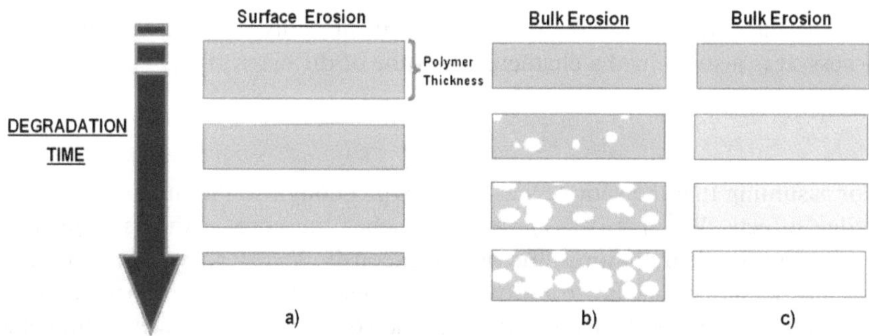

Fig. 4 Schematic illustration of three types of erosion phenomenon: (**a**) surface erosion, (**b**) bulk erosion with autocatalysis, (**c**) bulk erosion without autocatalysis (based on [54])

specimen. Polymers containing, ether, amide or ester groups, such as PLA, PGA, PCL, polyamide, proteins, and cellulose (and its derivatives), generally exhibit this type of erosion [34].

One other type is heterogeneous or surface erosion (Fig. 4a), in which hydrolysis occurs in the region near the surface, whereas the bulk material is only slightly or not hydrolyzed at all. As the surface is eroded and removed, the hydrolysis front moves through the material core. In this case, in which diffusion is very slow compared to hydrolysis, one must use Eq. (1) to calculate water concentration $w(t, x)$ at any instant t through the volume, before using Eqs. (8) or (9). The rate of boundary movement is very often nearly constant [27]. Surface eroding polymers have a greater ability to achieve zero-order release kinetics, i.e. a state at which the rate of an enzyme reaction is independent of the concentration of the substrate. Therefore, they are ideal candidates for developing devices able to deliver substances [32] such as drugs, growth factors, etc. Polymers such as poly(ortho ester)s (POEs), PAHs, and some polycarbonates tend to undergo surface erosion [54]. Also enzymatic erosion fits on this last type of erosion, since enzymes are unable to diffuse and present a raised hydrolysis kinetic constant k. In the presence of enzymes, heterogeneous hydrolytic damage can be modeled, considering a high hydrolysis kinetic constant k and a diffusion coefficient D close to zero. This damage should then be added to the damage due to water, either homogeneous or heterogeneous.

Surface and bulk erosion are ideal cases to which most polymers cannot be unequivocally assigned. Hence, two major processes have an impact on the erosion kinetics:

1. the diffusion of water into the polymer bulk, and
2. the hydrolytic degradation of the polymer backbone.

It is possible to define the characteristic time of hydrolysis, τ_H, as the inverse of hydrolysis rate [14]:

$$\tau_H = \frac{1}{kEw} = \frac{1}{u} \tag{12}$$

If D is the diffusion coefficient of water in the polymer and L is the sample thickness, it is also defined a characteristic time of diffusion, τ_D [14]:

$$\tau_D = \frac{L^2}{D} \tag{13}$$

For assuming that the sample surface is large enough so that it can be neglected the edge effects. When $\tau_H \gg \tau_D$, water reaches the core of the material before it reacts, and the degradation starts homogeneously. When $\tau_H \ll \tau_D$, water reacts totally in the superficial layer and will never reach the core of the material. The degradation starts heterogeneously through the volume. In these cases, a higher surface to volume ratio induces a faster degradation. So, in heterogeneous degradation fibers of smaller diameter will have, in average, a higher hydrolysis rate u than the larger diameter fibers. Critical conditions are defined when $\tau_D = \tau_H$. In this critical condition, the critical thickness can be defined as [14]:

$$L_c = \sqrt{\frac{D}{u}} \tag{14}$$

This critical thickness ranges from tens of micrometers for PAH's to a few centimeters for polyesters [14]. If the specimen thickness is larger than this critical size, the specimen undergoes surface erosion. Otherwise, it undergoes bulk erosion. Since diffusion and hydrolysis depend on temperature, pH of the aqueous media, etc., the critical thickness will depend on those parameters. According to Göpferich's point of view [14], all the water-insoluble degradable polymers could undergo surface erosion or bulk erosion at different conditions. In conclusion, the way a polymer matrix erodes depends on the diffusivity of water inside the matrix, the hydrolysis rate of the polymer's functional groups and the matrix dimensions. It should be noted that if laboratory experiments are carried out on samples with thickness lower than the critical value, they will not necessarily model thicker samples.

One factor that complicates the erosion is the autocatalytic hydrolysis reaction [38]. The hydrolytic degradation of aliphatic polyesters derived from lactic and glycolic acids (PLA/GA polymers) has been previously shown to proceed heterogeneously in the case of large size devices, the rate of degradation being greater inside than at the surface [16, 25, 50]. This was observed both *in vitro* [16] and *in vivo* [43]. For example, a thick plate of PLA erodes faster than a thinner one made of the same polymer [16]. This occurs due to retention of the oligomeric hydrolysis products within the material, unable to diffuse out if the material is very thick. These oligomeric reaction products are carboxylic acids, causing a decrease in pH and increased hydrofilicity in the core of the material, therefore accelerating locally the degradation [14] due to a local increase of hydrolysis kinetic constant, k.

As degradation proceeds, soluble oligomers which are close to the surface can leach out, whereas those which are located well inside the matrix remain entrapped and fully contribute to the autocatalytic effect. This difference of concentration in acidic groups, results in the formation of a skin composed of less degraded polymer. The thickness of this skin depends on many factors such as the diffusion rates of each involved species and the rate of ester bond cleavage. As can be seen in Fig. 4b, hollow structures are formed as a consequence [16]. A more complex model, with more parameters, is necessary to describe this phenomenon. This implies an extensive experimental characterization. However, this hollow formation occurs in the late stages of erosion, when molecular weight becomes greatly reduced. The models presented in the following section, to describe strength decrease and stress–strain plot evolution during degradation are only valid for the initial phase of erosion, i.e. for hydrolytic damage of about 50 %. Hence, these models neglect the hollow formation effect, since this phenomenon may be neglected during the first 50 % of strength loss, i.e. the mass loss and oligomer diffusion are neglected (as will be showed in the following sections).

Some authors claim that the local raise of degradation rate can also be explained by the local increase of hydrophilicity. The hydrophilicity involves the build-up of acid and alcohol groups, much more hydrophilic than the initial ester group [49]. An increasing water equilibrium concentration with time can thus be expected. It is quite simple to solve the problem, as Bellenger et al. [4] have shown, if it were considered, with Van Krevelen, that the water equilibrium concentration is an additive function, thus, $w = b + an_t$, and:

$$\frac{dC}{dt} = \frac{dn_t}{dt} = kE(C_0 + n_t)(b + an_t) \tag{15}$$

Solving Eq. (15), as demonstrated by Bellenger et al. [4], leads to:

$$n_r = C_0\left[\frac{b - aC_0}{be^{-kE(b-aC_0)t} - aC_0} - 1\right] \tag{16}$$

were a and b are material parameters. Accordingly to Bellenger et al. [4], this equation gives a good quantitative description of the auto-accelerated character of the degradation. If the auto-accelerated character is not due to increasing hydrophilicity, it is probably because its origin is in the hydrolysis mechanism. Alcohol groups and especially acid groups coming from the first degradation steps can catalyze later hydrolysis reactions.

7 Tuning Hydrolytic Rate According to Scaffold Requirements

To control the hydrolytic rate, in order to match the dimensioning requests during all the healing process, the project designer can combine different materials with different hydrolytic rates. A wide range of degradation times and mechanical properties are possible, using different commercial available materials and varying dimensions and 3D architecture. One possible approach is the composite concept, making use of the broad range of material properties to construct a multilayer device, each layer possessing its own degradation rate. The mixture law may also be applied to hydrolytic rate, assuming homogeneous degradation:

$$u_c = u_1 * V_1 + u_2 * V_2 + \cdots + u_i * V_i + \cdots + u_n * V_n = \sum_{i=1}^{n} u_n * V_n \tag{17}$$

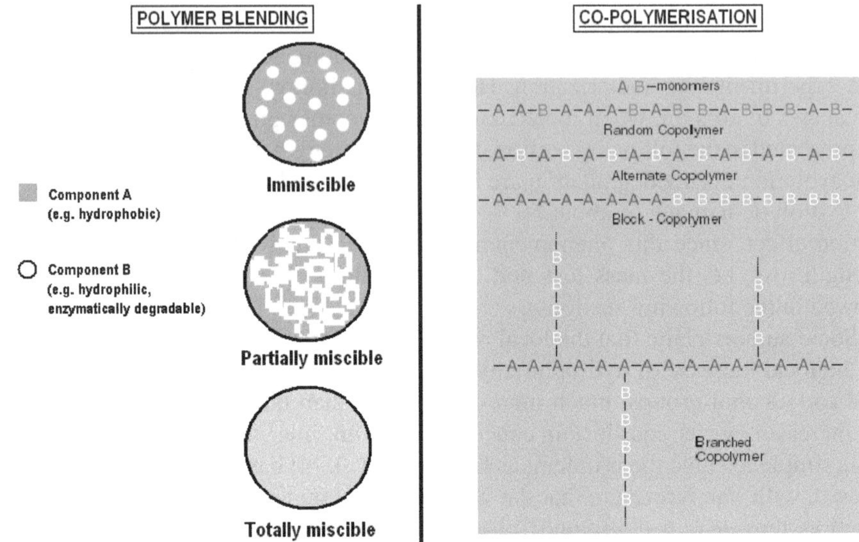

Fig. 5 Strategies to control degradation rate of biodegradable polymers

where V_i are the volume fractions of each material. Another way to control the hydrolytic rate constant of materials is by block copolymerization or blending with other biodegradable polymers, having different hydrolytic rate constants. Copolymers of several lactides or lactones can be synthesized by ring opening polymerization, resulting in high molecular weight polyesters [9]. The mixture of different polymers to produce blends, with controlled hydrolytic rate and mechanical properties can be performed in two ways: mixing the melted polymers, or mixing polymers solutions using a common solvent. However, the miscibility is limited, depending on polymers used and its volume fractions. The observation of two glass transition temperatures is a common way to evaluate immiscibility of the blends. In blends formulations with poor miscibility, the mixture of polymer solutions is preferable. Unfortunately, this solution implies the use of solvents, which have negative environmental effects. The different strategies to control degradation rate are represented in Fig. 5.

8 Characterization of Degradation Rate

The aim of this section is to demonstrate an example of experimental procedure to analyze erosion and degradation. Weight, strength and molecular weight evolutions were determined during degradation of polymers. At the end of this procedure, it was possible to determine the degradation rate u of the biodegradable material. In this example, and in the following sections, the material used is a blend of PLA-PCL (90:10). Two fiber dimensions were used (0.15 and 0.4 mm). Samples were placed

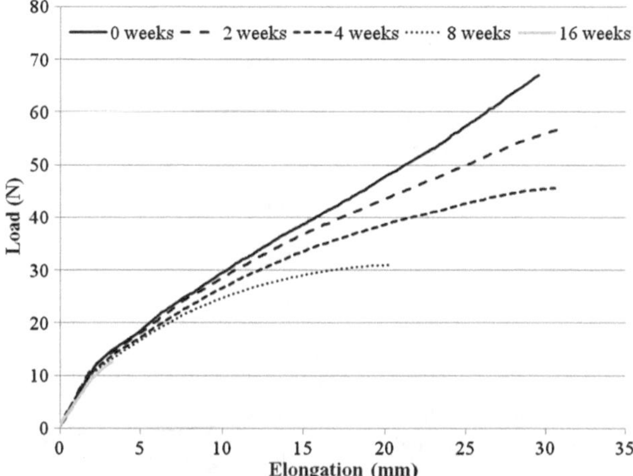

Fig. 6 Tensile test results for different degradation time of PLA-PCL fibers (400 μm) under PBS

in tubes and submitted to different degradation stages, under PBS (Phosphate Buffer Solution) at 37 °C. The duration of stages was previously determined, according to the supplier durability claims, until a maximum of 7 months. At the end of each degradation stage, pH of the media was measured, then test pieces were weighted after and before drying, further submitted to tensile tests and finally to GPC (Gel Permeation Chromatography) to measure molecular weight. The initial pH of the PBS solution was 8 (eight) and did not change significantly during degradation. As can be seen in Fig. 6, PLA-PCL has become brittle only after 16 weeks, lost its plasticity region, and strength has progressively decreased. The almost constant slope of the linear elastic stage indicates that no significant variation in Young modulus occurred during degradation.

For these PLA-PCL fibers, no significant differences were observed among the different dimensions tested, either in terms of strength and molecular weight evolutions during degradation (see Fig. 7). One can conclude that, in the present case, water diffusion can be assumed instantaneous and that hydrolysis takes place homogeneously throughout the samples (bulk degradation without autocatalysis) [2]. For highly heterogeneous degradation, the rate will not be globally similar, independently of dimensions, and the water concentration will locally depend on the position and time. As can be seen in Fig. 8, while in the first 16 weeks the fiber only looses 10 % of mass, it presents 80 % of strength loss.

From Fig. 9, one can see that the measured strength follows the same trend as the molecular weight, in a semi-logarithmic representation. The slope of this linear fitting, that includes all experimental results normalized to the initial value and in semi-logarithmic scale, represents the degradation rate. Instead of Eq. (8), a relationship similar to the one obtained for the molecular weight, Eq. (7), can be used,

$$\sigma = \sigma_0 e^{-u_s t} \tag{18}$$

where u_s is the strength decrease rate of the material. This parameter, u_s, seems to be directly related to the molecular weight decrease rate of the material, u_m, as can be

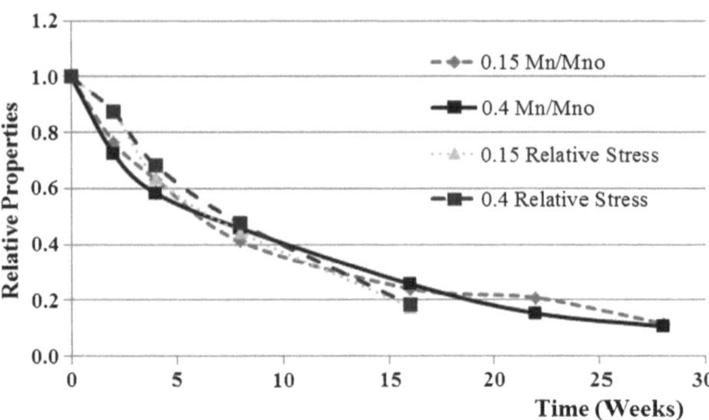

Fig. 7 Normalized: (a) strength and (b) molecular weight, for different degradation time of PLA-PCL fibers, of 150 μm and 400 μm, under PBS

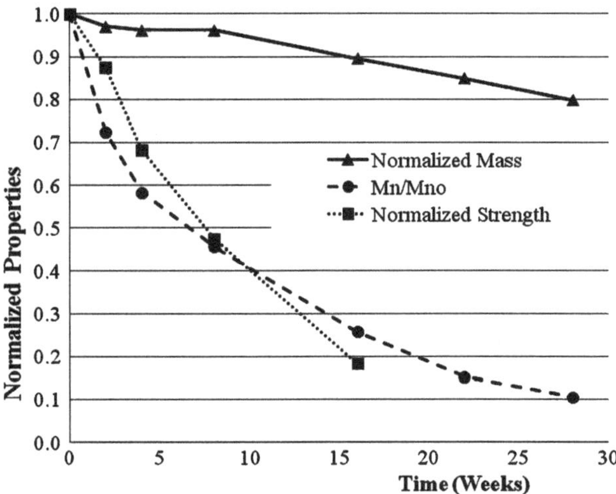

Fig. 8 Normalized: (a) mass, (b) molecular weight and strength, for different degradation time of PLA-PCL fibers, of 400 μm, under PBS

seen in Fig. 9 and in Table 1. This same trend can be found in the degradation results of other previous works, such as the one by Meek et al. [28], with PDLA-PCL. This can therefore provide a strategy to obtain a design failure criterion for the evolution of the limit strength of the device during the degradation process, $\sigma = f(t)$.

9 Constitutive Models to Simulate Mechanical Behavior During Hydrolytic Degradation

Whenever loading conditions are simple and the desired lifetime of mechanical support is known, a "trial and error" approach may be sufficient to design reasonable reliable devices. In more complex situations, scaffolds designers can use numerical approaches to define the material formulation and geometry that will satisfy the immediate needs of symptomatic relief. In these cases, they can use constitutive models supplied in the commercial packages of Finite Element Method (FEM) modeling, to simulate the mechanical behavior of a device in the most severe condition, based

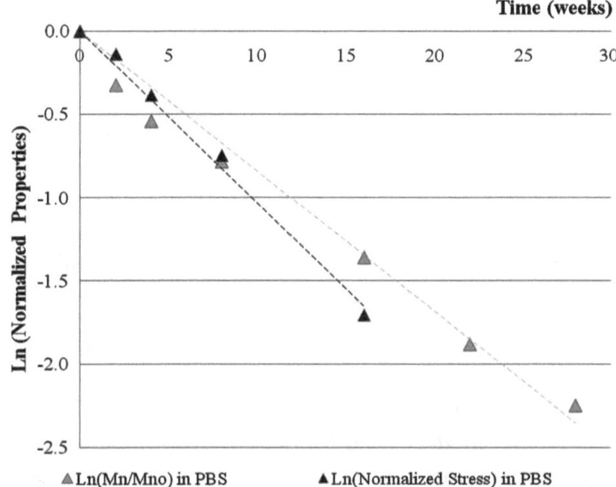

Fig. 9 Normalized strength and normalized molecular weight evolution for different degradation time of PLA-PCL fibers of 400 μm under PBS

on the initial material mechanical properties. However, the lack of design tools to predict long term behavior has limited the application of biodegradable materials.

A constitutive model for a mechanical analysis is a relationship between the response of a body (for example, strain state) and the stress state due to the forces acting on the body, which can include the environmental effects. A wide variety of material behaviors are described with a few different classes of constitutive equations. Mechanical properties of biodegradable plastics are commonly assessed within the scope of linearized elasticity, despite the clear evidence that they can undergo large strains before breaking. Due to the nonlinear nature of the stress vs, strain plot, the classical linear elastic model is clearly not valid for large strains simulation. Other plasticity or hyperelastic models are required to model those situations. Hence, given the nature of biodegradable polymers, classical models such as the Neo-Hookean and Mooney-Rivlin models, for incompressible hyperelastic materials, may be used to predict mechanical behavior until rupture of non-degraded PLA [13, 26]. A single-order, isotropic Ogden material hyperelastic model was also used [23] to simulate the mechanical behavior evolution during degradation of a polyester-urethane scaffold.

These models are useful to model the toughness of materials with this type of mechanical behavior. For these materials, the work assumption implies the existence of a scalar field, the stored energy function W, which is a function of the deformation gradient F. The stored energy function, W, can also be represented as a function of the right Cauchy–Green deformation tensor invariants. In general, the strain energy

Table 1 Degradation rate of PLA-PCL under PBS, determined by measuring strength and molecular weight evolution for different degradation time

	$Ln(\sigma/\sigma_o) = -u_s t$	R	$Ln(M_n/M_o) = -u_m t$	R
u	0.103	0.996	0.0841	0.989

density for an isotropic, incompressible, hyperelastic material is determined by two invariants. The first and second invariants in uniaxial tension are given by:

$$I_C = \lambda^2 + \frac{2}{\lambda} \tag{19}$$

$$II_C = \frac{1}{\lambda^2} + 2\lambda \tag{20}$$

where λ is the axial stretch ($\lambda = 1 + \varepsilon$), that satisfies $\lambda \geq 1$. For the Neo-Hookean incompressible hyperelastic solid, the stored energy function is given by:

$$W = \frac{\mu_1}{2}(I_C - 3) \tag{21}$$

where $\mu_1 > 0$ is the material property, usually called the shear modulus. An extension of this model is the Mooney-Rivlin incompressible hyperelastic solid, which stored energy function has the form:

$$W = \frac{\mu_1}{2}(I_C - 3) + \frac{\mu_2}{2}(II_C - 3) \tag{22}$$

with two material properties μ_1 and $\mu_2 > 0$. Higher order stored energy functions may be considered to describe the experimental data, such as a reduced 2nd order stored energy function, that includes a mixed term with both invariants of the right Cauchy–Green stretch tensor and an extra material constant μ_3, which the stored energy function has the form:

$$W = \frac{\mu_1}{2}(I_C - 3) + \frac{\mu_2}{2}(II_C - 3) + \frac{\mu_3}{6}(I_C - 3)(II_C - 3) \tag{23}$$

Considering the equations above, the axial nominal stress for the three models, Neo-Hookean (σ^{NH}), Mooney-Rivlin (σ^{MR}) and reduced second order ($\sigma^{2nd\,red}$), will be given by:

$$\sigma^{NH} = \mu_1\left(\lambda - \frac{1}{\lambda^2}\right) \tag{24}$$

$$\sigma^{MR} = \mu_1\left(\lambda - \frac{1}{\lambda^2}\right) + \mu_2\left(1 - \frac{1}{\lambda^3}\right) \tag{25}$$

$$\sigma^{2nd\,red} = (\mu_1 - \mu_3)\left(\lambda - \frac{1}{\lambda^2}\right) + (\mu_2 - \mu_3)\left(1 - \frac{1}{\lambda^3}\right) + \mu_3\left(\lambda^2 - \frac{1}{\lambda^4}\right) \tag{26}$$

According to Soares et al. [39], the model constitutive material parameters depend on degradation time. The material parameters are considered to be material functions of degradation damage instead of material constants. For fibers of a blend of PLA-PCL (90:10), it was determined that only the first material parameter μ_1 varies linearly with hydrolytic damage (as defined in Eq. (9)) [53].

From Fig. 10, one can see that the hyperelastic material models fit well the measured storage energy, for all the degradation steps up to 8 weeks (about 50 % of damage). The experimental data of storage energy was calculated by measuring

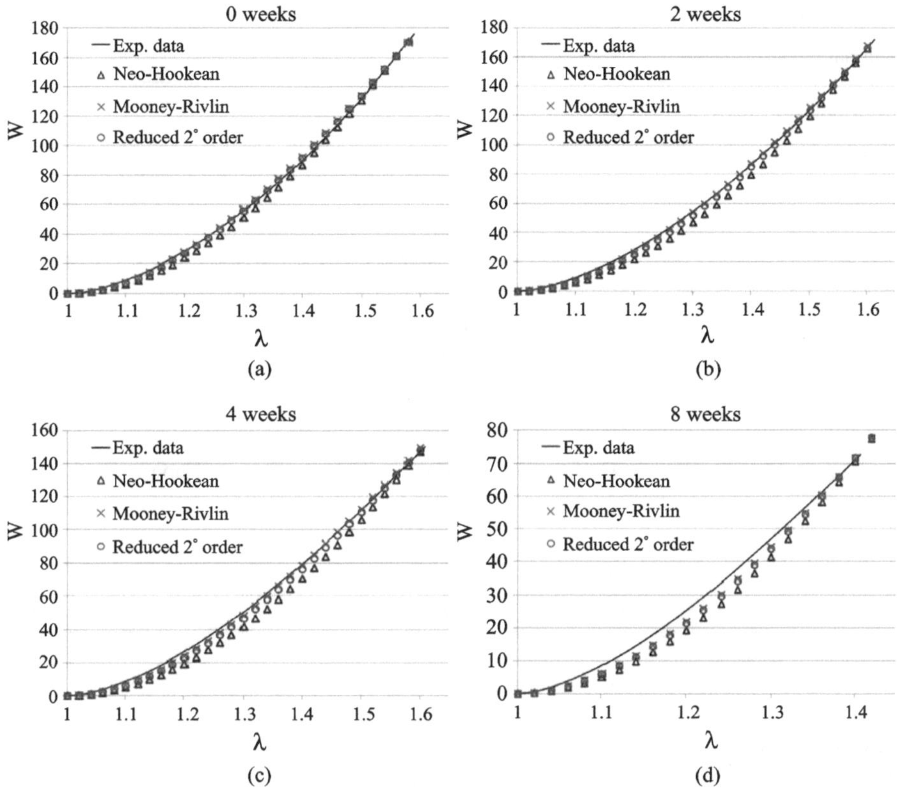

Fig. 10 Storage energy vs. axial stretch for 0, 2, 4 and 8 weeks of degradation [53]

the area (i.e., by taking the integral) underneath the stress-strain curve, from initial stretch (one) to the desired stretch level (no compression behavior was accessed). The Neo-Hookean model was the less accurate. However, it never violates the 2nd Law of Thermodynamics, which imposes that every material parameters μ_i must be positive. The material parameters were calculated by inverse parameterization based on the experimental data. The results are presented in Table 2.

If the last degradation stage is discarded, then the material model parameter, μ_1, varies linearly with the hydrolytic damage, as proposed by Soares et al. [39]. The proposed approach, which admits that only the first material parameter changes with hydrolytic damage, $\mu_1(d)$, according to the linear regressions (see Fig. 11), allows a good description of the mechanical behavior evolution, based on Eqs. (24), (25) or (26). Moreover the ultimate stress, which is the failure criterion used, can be defined by Eq. (18).

From Fig. 12, one can see that the hyper elastic material models allowed a reasonable approximation of the tensile test results, i.e. stress *vs* strain. However, the constitutive models are unable to describe precisely the initial elastic phase of the

Table 2 Material models parameters for different degradation time [53]

Material models	Weeks	D	μ_1	μ_2	μ_3
Neo-Hookean	0	0.00	450	–	–
	2	0.18	410		
	4	0.33	364		
	8	0.55	364		
	16	0.80	630		
Mooney-Rivlin	0	0.00	80	500	–
	2	0.18	50		
	4	0.33	5		
	8	0.55	−30		
	16	0.80	150		
2nd reduced order	0	0.00	155	400	−1
	2	0.18	120		
	4	0.33	75		
	8	0.55	50		
	16	0.80	250		

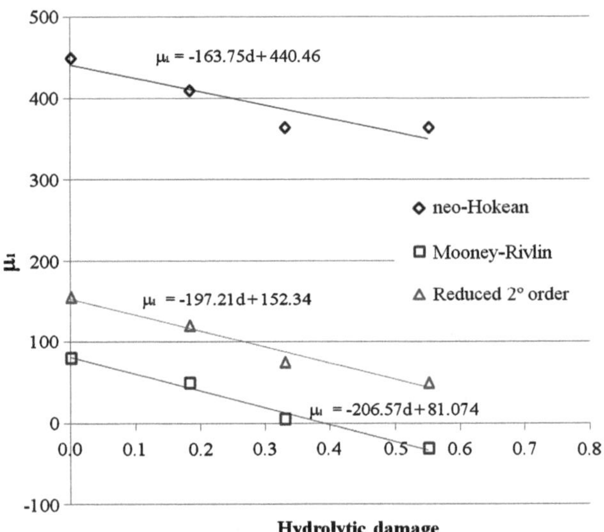

Fig. 11 Evolution of the material parameter, μ_1, for each model, considering different degradation time [53]

stress-strain plot, where the stiffness remains barely constant. This explains why the material model parameter, μ_1, increases sharply in the last degradation stage (16 weeks) for all three models, because the inverse parameterization was based on the experimental data that mostly comprehends elastic deformation.

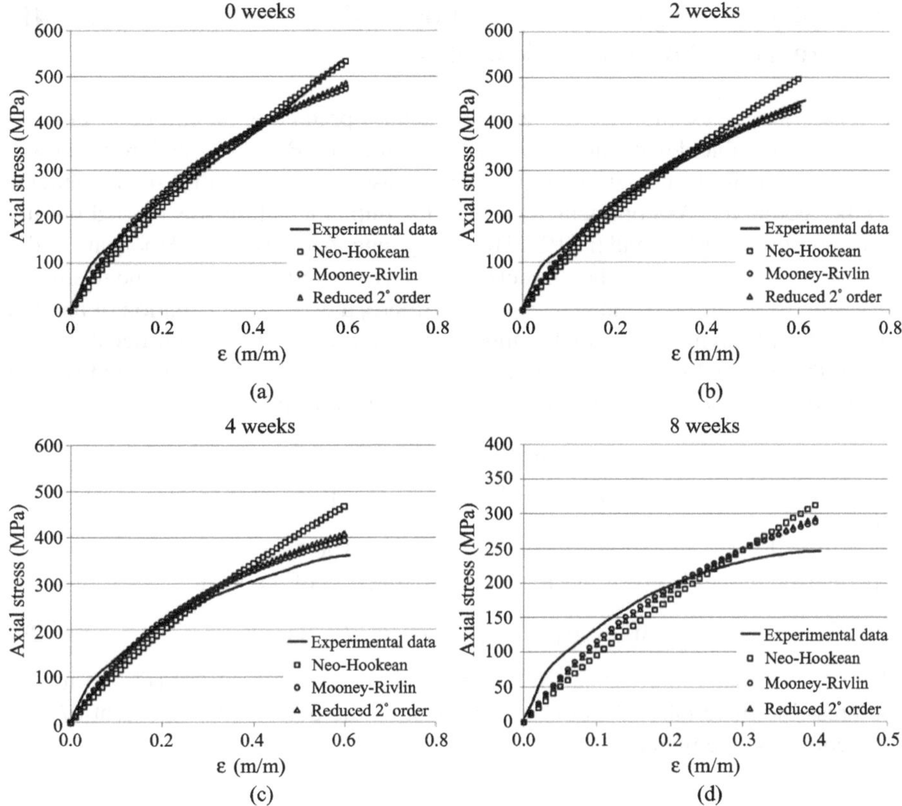

Fig. 12 Axial nominal stress vs. strain for 0, 2, 4 and 8 weeks of degradation (experimental data and material models) [53]

Tensile strength evolution can be determined during degradation in test specimens of PLA-PCL fibers or other elements with small thickness. This is possible since hydrolytic reaction is the limiting step of the overall degradation process. Diffusion may be neglected in these cases, and hydrolysis may be considered to take place homogeneously within the sample volume.

These constitutive models are available in commercial FEM software packages, but they are not linked to failure criterion. Thus, a new approach is proposed in which constitutive equations can be implemented in commercial FEM software packages like ABAQUS™, by changing the material parameter as function of hydrolytic damage or degradation time, and associated to the failure criterion implemented by a User Material (UMAT) subroutine, as well as PYTHON language. An example of this approach is given in the following section, for a simple geometry of a fiber.

10 Implementation and Application of the New Approach for 4D Numerical Analysis of Scaffolds

In this section, an example of the new approach for predicting the life-cycle of a hydrolytic degradable device, and its implementation in ABAQUS standard is shown, using the Neo-Hookean material model. This is used to simulate PLA-PCL behavior for fiber geometry. As commented earlier, this implementation was carried out using a subroutine UMAT and the PYTHON language. Although Neo-Hookean model was less accurate than the other models, it is not so complicate to implement, since it uses only one material parameter μ_1. Furthermore, it avoids the violation of the 2nd Law of Thermodynamics, which happens for the other models with negative values for the material parameters (μ_2 and μ_3). For this 3D case, the first and second invariants of deviator part of the left Cauchy-Green deformation tensor are given by:

$$I_{\mathrm{B}} = \mathrm{tr}(B) \tag{27}$$

$$II_B = 1/2\left[(\mathrm{tr}\,B)^2 - \mathrm{tr}\,B^2\right]^{1/2} \tag{28}$$

where B is the deviator stretch tensor ($B = FF^T$). The Neo-Hookean compressible hyper elastic model is given by stored energy function of the form:

$$W = (\mu_1/2)(I_B - 3) + G(J - 1)^2 \tag{29}$$

where G is a material constant that depends on the compressibility ($G = 0$ for incompressible materials). J is the determinant of the deformation gradient ($J = 1$ for incompressible materials):

$$J = \det(\partial x/\partial X) \tag{30}$$

where x is the current 3D position of a material point and X is the reference position of the same point. Then:

$$F = J^{-1/3}(\partial x/\partial X) \tag{31}$$

is the deformation gradient with volume change eliminated. The Cauchy stress tensor for the Neo-Hookean model used in this example is given by:

$$T = (\mu_1/J)\,\mathrm{dev}(B) + 2C(J - 1)I \tag{32}$$

where I is the 2nd order identity tensor.

The first material parameter is calculated as function of the hydrolytic damage, $\mu_1(d_h)$, according to a linear regression shown in Fig. 11.

In this example, a 3D model of a fiber was developed by means of a script in PYTHON language, using solid and axisymmetric elements, with parabolic interpolation functions, as well as with reduced and/or hybrid integration. This script is run by ABAQUS and the degradation time is required as an input parameter data (Fig. 13). The hydrolysis rate of the material (u) and the strength of the non-degraded material (σ_0) are initially set in the command lines. The material was considered nearly incompressible ($G = 10^{-3}$). Then the script calculates the hydrolytic damage (d_h) according to Eq. (9), and the material strength (σ_t) according to Eq. (8),

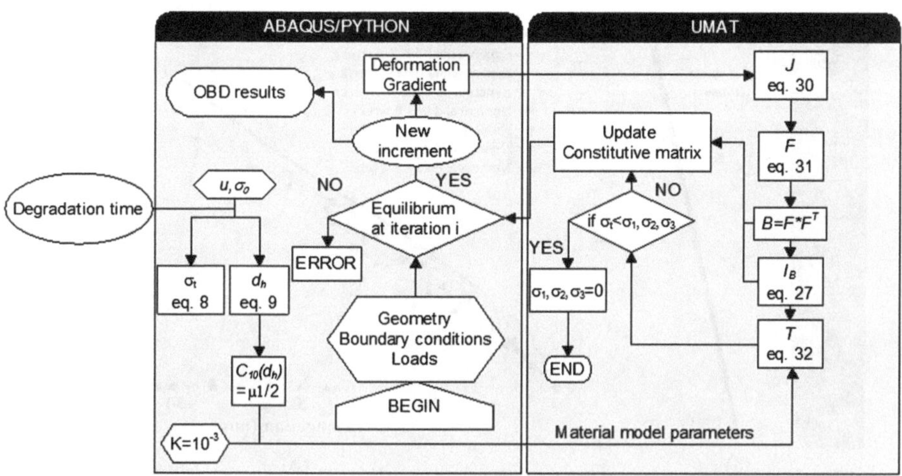

Fig. 13 Flow of operations done by ABAQUS/PYTHON and the UMAT subroutine [52]

for a given the degradation time (t). The script also calculates the material parameter ($C_{10} = \mu_1/2$) as a function of the hydrolytic damage $C_{10}(d_h)$. The material strength (σ_t) and the material parameters (C_{10} and G) are considered input data for the UMAT subroutine, as shown in Fig. 13.

Based on the geometry, the loadings and boundary conditions, ABAQUS calculates the variables that correspond to the deformation gradient ($\partial x/\partial X$). Then, the UMAT calculates the Jacobian (J) and the distortion tensor (F), according to Eqs. (30) and (31) respectively, for each integration point of the FEM model. The deviator stretch tensor B is then calculated before the calculation of stress Cauchy tensor T, according to Eq. (32). The implemented UMAT compares the principal stresses (σ_1, σ_2 and σ_3) to the strength (σ_t) for each integration point, acting as a failure criterion. Whenever these are greater than the strength, for a certain increment, the subroutine sets them to zero in the finite element analyzed. Finally, the UMAT constructs the constitutive matrix and calculates the result for each increment into the OBD (Output Base Data) file of ABAQUS. The flow chart of calculi operations is represented in Fig. 13.

Figure 14a shows the mesh of the finite element model and boundary conditions applied, as well as a numerical result for maximum principal stress. The CAX8H (8-node biquadratic axisymmetric quadrilateral, hybrid, linear pressure element) and C3D20RH (20-node quadratic brick, hybrid, linear pressure, reduced integration) element types were used, with similar results. Although the first element type is simpler and faster to calculate, it cannot be used in 3D complex shapes. From Fig. 14b, one can see that the hyper elastic material model allowed a reasonable approximation of the tensile test results reported previously. For this particular geometry and load conditions, no mesh size dependence was found. Finally, more details can be seen at Vieira et al. [52].

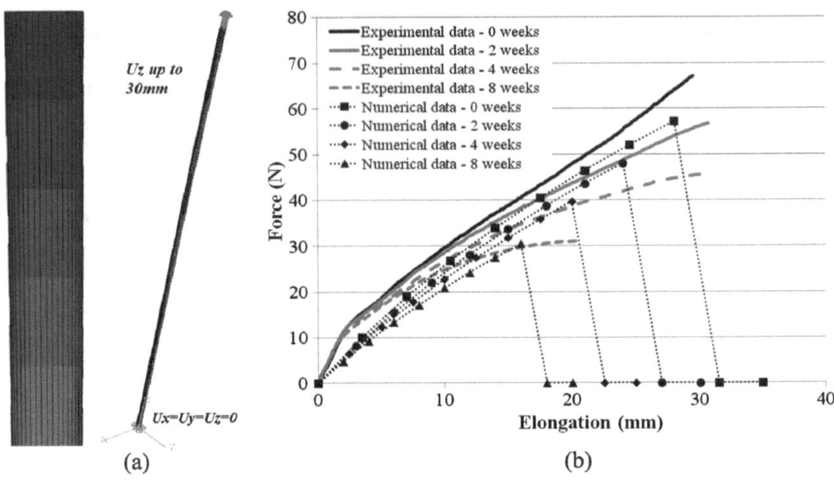

Fig. 14 (a) 3D model of the fiber; (b) Experimental vs. numerical results according of tensile tests to PLA-PCL fibers at different stages of hydrolytic degradation [52]

11 Conclusion

The numerical approach presented here can be used as design tool of biodegradable polymeric devices with further complex 3D geometries, considering the initial condition of instantaneous diffusion (homogeneous degradation along the volume). Although this approach was only tested with this particular blend, the authors believe that this can be extended to other thermoplastic biodegradable materials with response similar to hyper elastic behavior. For example, presently 3D scaffolds can be printed with biodegradable polymers. Using this new approach, complex geometries can be modeled in a commercial 3D drawing software, or digitalized from biomedical images, and then exported to ABAQUS™ to predict its mechanical behavior during degradation by numerical simulation. This approach, only valid for small thickness devices in the first steps of erosion, without considering the degradation rate dependence on temperature, environment and stress state, can be further expanded to more detailed models that consider these dependencies, the crystalline degree dependence, and the diffusion of water, enzymes and degradation products. In these further complex problems, damage will depend not only on the degradation time, but also on the water concentration and the hydrolysis kinetic constant, no longer constants but time, geometrical, degradation media, temperature and stress state dependents.

The development of better models for biodegradable polymers can enhance the scaffolds design process. The numerical approach presented here, based on the calculation of one material parameter of Neo-Hookean hyper elastic model, that is a function of the degradation time, can overcome this limitation and enable a reasonably prediction of the life time of newer and more complex scaffolds.

Acknowledgements The authors Vieira A. and Guedes R.M. would like to thank the FCT (Portuguese Science and Technology Foundation) for financial support under the grants PTDC/EME-PME/70155/2006 and PTDC/EME-PME/114808/2009. Tita V. would like to thank FAPESP (Research Foundation of State of São Paulo) for financial support under the grant 09/00544-5. The authors would like to highlight that this work was also partially supported by the Program USP/UP, which is a scientific cooperation agreement established between the University of Porto (Portugal) and the University of São Paulo (Brazil).

References

1. Aslan S, Calandrelli L, Laurienzo P, Malinconico M, Migliares C (2000) Poly(d,l-lactic ac-id)/poly(caprolactone) blend membranes: preparation and morphological characterization. J Mater Sci 35:1615–1622
2. Auras R, Harte B, Selke S (2004) An overview of polylactides as packaging materials. Macromol Biosci 4:835–864
3. Bastin G, Dochain D (1990) On-line estimation and adaptive control of bioreactor. Elsevier, Amsterdam
4. Bellenger V, Ganem M, Mortaigne B, Verdu J (1995) Lifetime prediction in the hydrolytic age-ing of polyesters. Polym Degrad Stab 49:91–97
5. Bikiaris D, Papageorgiou G, Achilias D, Pavlidou E, Stergiou A (2007) Miscibility and enzymatic degradation studies of poly(e-caprolactone)/poly(propylene succinate) blends. Eur Polym J 43:2491–2503
6. Chen G-Q, Wu Q (2005) Review: the application of polyhydroxyalkanoates as tissue engineering materials. Biomaterials 26:6565–6578
7. Chu CC (1985) Strain-accelerated hydrolytic degradation of synthetic absorbable sutures. In: Hall CW (ed) Surgical research, recent developments: proceedings of the first annual scientific session of the Academy of Surgical Research. Pergamon Press, San Antonio
8. Colombo A, Karvouni E (2000) Biodegradable stents: fulfilling the mission and stepping away. Circulation 102:371–373
9. Endo M, Aida T, Inoue A (1987) Immortal polymerization of e-caprolactone initiated by aluminum porphyrin in the presence of alcohol. Macromolecules 20:2982–2988
10. Fan LT, Lee Y (1983) Kinetic studies of enzymatic hydrolysis of insoluble cellulose: derivation of a mechanistic kinetic model. Biotechnol Bioeng 25:2707–2733
11. Fan LT, Lee Y, Beardmore DH (1980) Major chemical and physical features of cellulosic materials as substrates for enzymatic hydrolysis. Adv Biochem Eng 14:101–117
12. Farrar DF, Gilson RK (2002) Hydrolytic degradation of polyglyconate B: the relationship between degradation time, strength and molecular weight. Biomaterials 23:3905–3912
13. Garlotta DA (2001) Literature review of poly(latic acid). J Polym Environ 9:63–84
14. Göpferich A (1996) Mechanisms of polymer degradation and erosion. Biomaterials 17:103–114
15. Göpferich A, Langer R (1993) Modeling of polymer erosion. Macromolecules 26:4105–4112
16. Grizzi I, Garreau H, Li S, Vert M (1995) Hydrolytic degradation of devices based on poly[DL-lactic acid size-dependence. Biomaterials 16:305–311
17. Han X, Pan J (2009) A model for simultaneous crystallization and biodegradation of biodegradable polymers. Biomaterials 30:423–430
18. Herzog K, Müller R-J, Deckwer W-D (2006) Mechanism and kinetics of the enzymatic hydrolysis of polyester nanoparticles by lipases. Polym Degrad Stab 91:2486–2498
19. Hill CG (1977) An introduction to chemical engineering kinetics and reactor design. Wiley, New York
20. Kennedy JF, Melo EHM (1990) Bioconversions of cellulose—a major source of material for the biochemical industry. Br Polym J 23:193–198

21. Kirby AJ (1972) Hydrolysis and formation of esters of organic acids. In: Bamford CH, Tipper CFH (eds) Comprehensive chemical kinetics, ester formation and hydrolysis and related reactions. Elsevier, Amsterdam

22. Klyosov AA, Rabinowitch M (1980) Enzymatic conversion of cellulose to glucose: present state of the art and potential. Plenum Press, New York

23. Krynauw H, Bruchmüller L, Bezuidenhout D, Zilla P, Franz T (2011) Constitutive modelling of degradation induced mechanical changes in a polyester-urethane scaffold for soft tissue regeneration. In: Fernandes PR et al (eds) Proceedings of II international conference on tissue engineering. Lisbon

24. Levenberg S, Langer R (2004) Advances in tissue engineering. In: Schatten GP (ed) Current topics in developemental biology. Elsevier, San Diego

25. Li SM, Garreau H, Vert M (1990) Structure-property relationships in the case of the degradation of massive aliphatic poly(α-hydroxyacids) in aqueous media. Part 3: Influence of the morphology of poly(L-lactic acid). J Mater Sci, Mater Med 1:198–206

26. Lunt J (1998) Large-scale production, properties and applications of polylatic acid polymers. Polym Degrad Stab 59:145–152

27. Lyu SP, Sparer R, Untereker D (2005) Analytical solutions to mathematical models of the surface and bulk erosion of solid polymers. J Polym Sci, Part B 43:383–397

28. Meek M, Jansen K, Steendam R, van Oeveren W, van Wachem P, van Luyn M (2004) In vitro degradation and biocompatibility of poly(DL-lactide-ε-caprolactone) nerve guides. J Biomed Mater Res, Part A 68:43–51

29. Metzmacher I, Radu F, Bause M, Knabner P, Friess W (2007) A model describing the effect of enzymatic degradation on drug release from collagen minirods. Eur J Pharm Biopharm 67:349–360

30. Miller ND, Williams DF (1984) The in vivo and in vitro degradation of poly(glycolic acid) suture material as a function of applied strain. Biomaterials 5:365–368

31. Morrison RT, Boyd RN (1992) Organic chemistry. Prentice Hall, New Jersey

32. Nair LS, Laurencin CT (2007) Biodegradable polymers as biomaterials. Prog Polym Sci 32:762–798

33. Nikolic MS, Poleti D, Djonlagic J (2003) Synthesis and characterization of biodegradable poly(butylene succinate-co-butylene fumarate)s. Eur Polym J 39:2183–2192

34. Pitt GG, Gratzl MM, Kimmel GL, Surles J, Sohindler A (1982) Aliphatic polyesters II. The degradation of poly(d,l-lactide), poly(e-caprolactone), and their copolymers in vivo. Biomaterials 2:215–220

35. Saha SK, Tsuji H (2009) Enhanced crystallization of poly(L lactide-co-ε caprolactone) in the presence of water. J Appl Polym Sci 112:715–720

36. Seretoudi G, Bikiaris D, Panayiotou C (2002) Synthesis, characterization and biodegradability of poly(ethylene succinate)/poly(e-caprolactone) block copolymers. Polymer 43:5405–5415

37. Shen-Guo W, Bo Q (1992) Polycaprolactone–poly(ethylene glycol) block copolymer, I: Synthesis and degradability in vitro. Polym Adv Technol 4:363–368

38. Siparsky GL, Voorhees KJ, Miao F (1998) Hydrolysis of polylactic acid (PLA) and polycaprolactone (PCL) in aqueous acetonitrile solutions: autocatalysis. J Environ Polym Degrad 6:31–41

39. Soares JS, Rajagopal KR, Moore JE (2010) Deformation induced hydrolysis of a degradable polymeric cylindrical annulus. Biomech Model Mechanobiol 9:177–186

40. Södergard A, Stolt M (2002) Properties of lactic acid based polymers and their correlation with composition. Prog Polym Sci 27:1123–1163

41. Sykes P (1975) A guidebook to mechanism in organic chemistry. Longman, London

42. Tamela TL, Talja M (2003) Biodegradable urethral stents. BJU Int 92:843–850

43. Therin M, Christel P, Li SM, Garreau H, Vert M (1992) In vivo degradation of massive poly(a-hydroxyacids): validation of in vitro findings. Biomaterials 13:594–600

44. Tokiwa Y, Suzuki T (1977) Hydrolysis of polyesters by lipase. Nature 270:76–78

45. Tsuji H, Ikada Y (1998) Properties and morphology of poly(L-lactide). II. Hydrolysis in alkaline solution. J Polym Sci, Part A 36:59–66

46. Tsuji H, Ikada Y (2000) Properties and morphology of poly(L-lactide) 4. Effects of structural parameters on long-term hydrolysis of poly(L-lactide) in phosphate-buffered solution. Polym Degrad Stab 67:179–189
47. Tsuji H, Nakahara K (2001) Poly(L-lactide)—IX hydrolysis in acid media. J Appl Polym Sci 86:186–194
48. Tzafriri AR, Bercovier M, Parnas H (2002) Reaction diffusion model of enzymatic erosion of insoluble fibrillar matrices. Biophys J 83:776–793
49. Van Krevelen DW (1976) Properties of polymers. Elsevier, Amsterdam
50. Vert M, Li S, Garreau H (1991) More about the degradation of LA/GA-derived matrices in aqueous media. J Control Release 16:15–26
51. Vieira AC, Guedes RM, Marques AT (2009) Development of ligament tissue biodegradable devices: a review. J Biomech 42:2421–2430
52. Vieira AC, Marques AT, Guedes RM, Tita V (2011) Material model proposal for biodegradable materials. Proc Eng 10:1597–1602
53. Vieira AC, Vieira JC, Ferra JM, Magalhães FD, Guedes RM, Marques AT (2011) Mechanical study of PLA–PCL fibres during in vitro degradation. J Mech Behav Biomed 4:451–460
54. von Burkersroda F, Schedl L, Göpferich A (2002) Why biodegradable polymers undergo surface or bulk erosion. Biomaterials 23:4221–4231
55. Walker LP, Wilson DB (1991) Enzymatic hydrolysis of cellulose: an overview. Bioresour Technol 36:3–14
56. Wang Y, Pan J, Han X, Sinka C, Ding L (2008) A phenomenological model for the degradation of biodegradable polymers. Biomaterials 29:3393–3401
57. Ward I (1983) Mechanical properties of solid polymers. Wiley, Chichester
58. Yu R, Chen H, Chen T, Zhou X (2008) Modeling and simulation of drug release from multilayer biodegradable polymer microstructure in three dimensions. Simul Model Pract Theory 16:15–25
59. Zhang X, Espiritu M, Bilyk A, Kurniawan L (2008) Morphological behaviour of poly(lactic acid) during hydrolytic degradation. Polym Degrad Stab 93:1964–1970

Microrheology of Biopolymers at Non-thermal Regimes

Rommel G. Bacabac, Heev Ayade, Lara Gay M. Villaruz, Raymund Sarmiento, and Roland Otadoy

Abstract Many studies demonstrate the relevance of the mechanical properties of molecules and living cells to physiological function. Therefore, several techniques have been developed to probe the rheology of biological materials. Among them are based on the analysis of embedded probe fluctuations. However, novel applications using this robust tool are still lacking, despite the fact that the study of living matter routinely demonstrate new phenomena, not immediately characterized by existing analytical tools developed in physics. Hence, we derive novel robust tools to adapt ways of probing non-linear and non-equilibrium phenomena for biological samples. We propose designs of optical tweezer systems using two-beam tandems by dual-wavelength and single-wavelength splitting, for the study of microrheology in bulk down to single biopolymer or protein based on the fluctuation spectra of embedded or attached probes. We generalize, for the first time, calculations for winding turn probabilities to account for unfolding events in single fibrous biopolymers, which is modeled using a newly derived worm-like-chain model re-expressed by fractional strain expansion. The ensuing probe fluctuations are taken as originating from a damped harmonic oscillator. The approach described here offer new ways of characterizing biopolymer rheology using parameters based on folding turns and a newly derived WLC expansion for non-linear stretching.

1 Introduction

Several recent results demonstrate the relevance of mechanics to biological function. Recently, Discher et al. have shown that cells grown on substrates of specific stiffness influence the differentiation lineage, which becomes irreversible after a long period of culture [1, 2]. We measured the elastic properties of bone cells (modeled

R.G. Bacabac (✉) · H. Ayade · L.G.M. Villaruz
Medical Biophysics Group, Department of Physics, University of San Carlos, Nasipit, Talamban, Cebu City 6000, Philippines
e-mail: rgbacabac@gmail.com

R. Sarmiento · R. Otadoy
Materials Physics Group, Department of Physics, University of San Carlos, Cebu City, Philippines

P.R. Fernandes, P.J. Bártolo (eds.), *Tissue Engineering,*
Computational Methods in Applied Sciences 31, DOI 10.1007/978-94-007-7073-7_5,
© Springer Science+Business Media Dordrecht 2014

using MLO-Y4 cells) and correlated these with their ability to release nitric oxide in response to minute stresses; we showed that cell shape directly correlated with the measured elastic modulus and mechanosensitivity [3], supporting the notion that physical parameters drive biologically relevant functions [4–7]. However, the underlying biophysical events are not well understood. Among several hypotheses, one may associate molecule-level deformation of trans-membrane proteins on cell membranes as triggering event to initiate relevant biochemical cascades directly affecting cell behavior [4, 8, 9]. Although promising, corresponding models for complex molecule deformation is still lacking. An approach based on approximating molecules as elastic rods are particularly successful in assessing high frequency fluctuations of biopolymers (at thermal equilibrium) [10–14]. However, biopolymers have complex structures [15–17], which have unknown coupling to their mechanical properties, and trans-membrane proteins are subjected to non-thermal forces at the onset of mechanosensing. Therefore, to develop a generic and robust approach, this study aims to design experimental and analytical methods for quantifying helical biopolymer deformation, since the helix is a basic structure from which higher orders of structure could be based.

A simple molecular geometry with sufficient complexity is that of a helix. Deoxyribonucleic acid, or DNA follows a helical structure and under right conditions form higher order coils that may appear globular. Actin, one of the cytoskeletal proteins, is also a helix, whereas collagen, a common tissue biopolymer is a triple helix [15, 16]. A previous study from Bernido and Carpio-Bernido 2005 showed that protein folding can be characterized using winding probabilities associated with the number of turns and the resulting length of the biopolymer under the appropriate strain [18, 19]. This approach is here adapted and will be investigated for characterizing biopolymer tension based on the unwinding of its helical structure under pre-defined tension.

A robust experimental tool for measuring the mechanical properties of molecules to living cells uses colloidal particles as probes. The Brownian motion of an embedded probe could be used to infer the complex shear modulus to quantify bulk mechanical properties of soft materials (e.g., a living mammalian cell) [11, 20–22]. In single biopolymers, the fluctuation spectra of an attached probe contain enough information to quantify mechanical properties. A low-cost optical trap system can be implemented in microscopes (in bright field or differential interference contrast mode) to manipulate and monitor the Brownian motion of optically confined probes for one-particle or two-point passive microrheology [3, 20, 21, 23–25]. Active microrheology is however implemented by measuring the mechanical responses to stimulation by wiggling a trapped embedded probe at known oscillations.

2 The Winding Probability Function

Depending on a single biopolymer's stiffness, its mechanical properties can be fully described based on a few parameters. For example, very compliant polymers could be described using its persistence length (e.g., deoxyribonucleic acid or DNA molecules) whereas semi-flexible polymers (e.g., actin or microtubules) could be described by monitoring bending fluctuations along its length [10, 26–28]. To find a more robust description that may start without a priori knowledge of the biopolymer's stiffness, the inferred properties could be based on the biopolymer's structure. In order to experimentally test this approach, the fluctuation of attached probes could be monitored and analyzed based only on the resulting length and winding turns of the biopolymer under known tensile strength.

Considering solutions to the Fokker-Plank equation, the probability density is derived using Feynman path integrals as possible conformations of a biopolymer. Specific to helical conformations, we derive the winding probability $W(n)$ about its longitudinal axis [18, 19] as follows:

$$W(n, L) = R\sqrt{\frac{4\pi}{Ll}} \frac{\exp\left[-\frac{R^2}{Ll}(2\pi n + \frac{l}{2DR}\int_0^L f(s)\,ds)^2\right]}{\theta_3\left(\frac{l}{4DR}\int_0^L f\,ds\right)} \tag{1}$$

where D is a constant drift coefficient, and the following parameters descriptive of the biopolymer: R = helical radius, L = total length, l = subunit length (such that $L = Nl$, N = number of sub-units or monomers in the biopolymer, $n = \pm 1, \pm 2, \pm 3, \ldots$, the total number of turns, clockwise ($-$) or counter-clockwise ($+$)). Here, $f(s)$ is to be understood as the drift coefficient of each sub-unit. Thus, if there were N total sub-units, we have $f_1, f_2, \ldots$ quantify the drift along the length of the biopolymer as the sum of the drift about each sub-unit:

$$F_f = \int_0^L f(s)\,ds \cong \sum_{m=1}^{N} f_m(\Delta s) \tag{2}$$

the theta function is:

$$\theta_3(u) = 1 + 2\sum_{m=1}^{\infty} q^{m^2}\cos(2mu)$$

$$u = \frac{l}{4DR}\int f(s)\,ds \tag{3}$$

$$q = \exp\left(-Ll/4R^2\right)$$

Note however, where we have a long biopolymer, $Nl \gg 1$, the theta function approaches unity, $\theta_3 \approx 1$. In this model the drift coefficient $f(s)$ is predicted to modulate the final conformation of the biopolymer in question. Thus, by choosing an approximate formulation of $f(s)$ or F_f, the conformation is predicted in terms only of winding-times (n) and the total length after stretching L. Note however that elastic moduli are not explicitly incorporated in this approach, which at first instance, could be considered implicit in $f(s)$. Since the winding probability $W(n, L)$ is both a function of n and L, the experimental approach involves stretching (variation in L) and counting winding (variations in n). Thus, the winding probability $W(n, L)$ captures a biopolymer's conformational adaptation based on the number of windings n, and the measured length L.

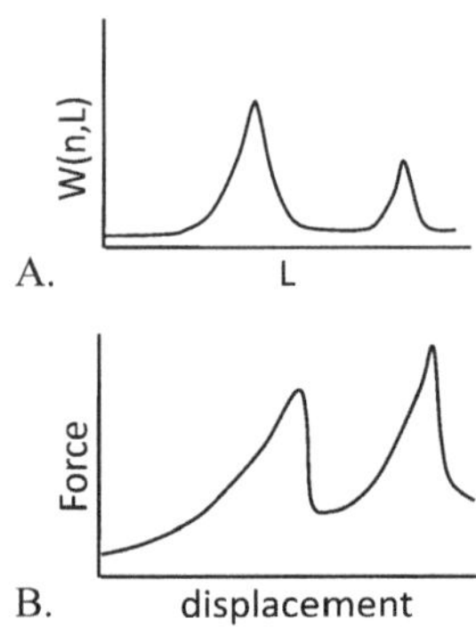

Fig. 1 Winding probability as events of unfolding. **A.** The model by Bernido et al. [18, 19] is here generalized to indicate probabilities of unfolding events at given length L, and a generalized event count designated by variable n. **B.** Hypothetical force-displacement curve in unfolded proteins responding to constant force application

The above theoretical tool was used for predicting known folding structures of real proteins [19]. Here we generalize this analytical tool and instead consider the variable n as events of unfolding (with L still designating the length; Fig. 1A). Consider that a hypothetical force-displacement curve for unfolding proteins stretched by force (using optical tweezers or atomic force microscopy) would show peaks that indicate stiffening and force collapse indicating a transition to the next structural unit. Since stiffening and force collapse are events when proteins resist unfolding and soften between unfolding events, our generalization for the use of variable n becomes natural. Note however that the winding probability, $W(n, L)$, and the force-displacement curves are not similarly symmetric. This, we account to the fact that the force directions are opposite at stiffening and softening events during the unfolding of a stretched biopolymer.

3 Non-linear Stretching of Biopolymers

The properties of stretched semi-flexible biopolymers are essentially captured by the worm-like-chain (WLC) model, which allows for an approximation of the force-extension relation:

$$F = \frac{k_B T}{L_p}\left[\frac{1}{4}\left(1 - \frac{\delta}{L}\right)^2 + \frac{\delta}{L} - \frac{1}{4}\right] \tag{4}$$

where the applied force, F, is based on the temperature, T, the Boltzmann constant, k_B, the contour length, L, the persistence length, L_p, and the small extension, δ due to the applied force. However, the WLC model does not include non-thermal conditions. Thus, to include non-linear effects at forces beyond thermal equilibrium magnitudes, we derived a new expression by fractional strain expansion (not demonstrated here):

$$F = \frac{k_B T}{L_p}\sum_{n=0}^{N_{WLC}}\left[\left(\frac{3}{p^2}\right)^{n+1}\left(\frac{\delta}{L_p}\right)^n\right] \tag{5a}$$

$$L = p L_p \tag{5b}$$

where the applied force, F, is expressed in terms of the fractional strain, δ/L_p, and a scaling parameter, p, which relates the contour length to the persistence length. Here, the order of expansion is truncated to N_{WLC}, where the force-extension relation fits experimental data.

Together with the winding probability, the scaling parameter, p, and both the number of turns and order of expansion (WLC fractional strain expansion order) offer novel ways of characterizing an over-stretched biopolymer. Whereas, the winding probability may be useful for predicting biopolymer folding (where fluid drag along the biopolymer length is implicit in $f(s)$), our newly derived WLC expansion implicitly incorporates material properties (via persistence length and fractional strain-force relations), where N_{WLC} can be interpreted as characteristic number.

4 Microrheology

The mechanical properties of a soft material at microscopic scales can be measured by wiggling a colloidal probe embedded (*active microrheology*) or by monitoring the thermal fluctuations of the probe (*passive microrheology*) [29]. To derive expressions for measuring mechanical properties, the apparent compliance, $\alpha(\omega)$, is here defined as the ratio of the amplitude of the bead displacement to the applied force:

$$\alpha(\omega) = \frac{u(\omega)}{f_d(\omega)} \tag{6}$$

Noting that the Stoke's law relates the drag force, f_d, on a moving sphere of velocity v (with radius R_s) to the fluid's viscosity, η:

$$f_d = 6\pi R_s \eta v \tag{7}$$

this recalls Newton's law for viscous fluids, where the shear stress σ is proportional to the rate of strain $d\gamma/dt$ as follows:

$$f_d/6\pi R_s = \eta v \quad \Rightarrow \quad \sigma \propto \eta \frac{d\gamma}{d}t \tag{8}$$

This expression, we generalize while assuming that the particle is dragged through a viscoelastic medium, such that $G''/(\omega) \sim \eta$ ($G^* = G' + iG''$, the complex shear modulus). Thus, instead of the drag force we now speak of stress in the material and find an expression for the shear modulus, G, with the velocity, du/dt (from (4)):

$$f_d = 6\pi R_s \frac{G}{\omega} v = 6\pi R_s G \frac{1}{\omega}\left(\frac{du}{dt}\right) \quad \Rightarrow \quad f_d\, dt = 6\pi R_s \frac{G}{\omega} du \tag{9}$$

from here we continue by integrating as follows (where f_d is sinusoidal):

$$\int f_d \omega\, dt = \int df_d = 6\pi R_s G \int du$$

$$\Rightarrow \quad f_d = 6\pi R_s G u \quad \Rightarrow \quad \frac{u(\omega)}{f_d(\omega)} = \frac{1}{6\pi R_s G(\omega)} \tag{10}$$

5 One Particle Active Microrheology

Since the applied force f is sinusoidal, its differential replaces: $f_d \omega\, dt \to df_d$ and G is expressed by the ratio of u to f in the frequency domain. From (6) and (10) we arrive at the generalized Stokes-Einstein relation (GSER) [22, 23], which shows how the complex shear modulus G^* is calculated from the probe response and the complex compliance α^*, in the frequency domain [21, 22]:

$$\alpha^*(\omega) = \frac{1}{6\pi R_s G^*(\omega)} \tag{11}$$

where the real and imaginary components refer to the elastic and viscous properties, respectively.

6 One Particle Passive Microrheology

From the Fluctuation-dissipation theory (FDT), the viscous compliance, $\alpha''(\omega)$, is related to the power spectral density $C(\omega)$:

$$\alpha''(\omega) = \frac{\omega}{4k_B T} C(\omega) \tag{12a}$$

where k_B is the Boltzmann constant and T is the absolute temperature. The elastic compliance, $\alpha'(\omega)$, is then calculated via the Kramers-Kronig relation from Linear Response Theory:

$$\alpha'(\omega) = \frac{2}{\pi} P \int_0^\infty \frac{\omega' \alpha''(\omega')}{\omega'^2 - \omega}\, d\omega' \tag{12b}$$

where P refers to the *Cauchy principal value* calculation. As shown earlier, the complex shear modulus is calculated from (11).

7 Two-Point Active Microrheology

So far we have derived expressions for calculating $G^*(\omega)$ by manipulating a single probe or by monitoring its thermal fluctuations. This method measures local viscoelastic properties surrounding the single probe. However, by extending the measurement using two identical probes, the bulk properties of the intervening material can be determined. Denoting the displacement responses of the first and second probes as u_1 and u_2, respectively, to the applied forces, f_2 and f_1, on the corresponding opposite probes, the mutual compliance of the intervening material is calculated by *two-point active microrheology* as [21]:

$$\alpha_{12}(\omega) = \frac{u_1(\omega)}{f_2(\omega)} \tag{13a}$$

$$\alpha_{21}(\omega) = \frac{u_2(\omega)}{f_1(\omega)} \tag{13b}$$

$$\alpha_{12}(\omega) = \alpha_{21}(\omega) \tag{13c}$$

where the displacements and applied forces are parallel. Note that the compliance is the same (13c) regardless of the order of the paired stimulus-response (force-displacement) measurements, assuming homogeneity in the sample.

8 Two-Point Passive Microrheology

At thermal equilibrium, the parallel cross-correlations of paired probes are monitored to measure the corresponding apparent viscous mutual compliance $\alpha_{12}''(\omega)$ [21]:

$$\alpha_{12}''(\omega) = \frac{\omega}{4k_B T} \langle u_1(\omega)u_2(\omega) \rangle \tag{14}$$

We then use the *Kramers-Kronig* integration to calculate the apparent elastic mutual compliance, $\alpha_{12}'(\omega)$:

$$\alpha_{12}'(\omega) = \frac{2}{\pi} \mathrm{P} \int_0^\infty \frac{\omega' \alpha_{12}''(\omega')}{\omega'^2 - \omega} \, d\omega' \tag{15}$$

The mutual complex shear modulus by *active* or *passive* mode, is calculated from the *parallel* mutual compliance (based on parallel displacements between probes):

$$G_{12}(\omega) = \frac{1}{4\pi r_{12}\alpha_{12}^{\|}(\omega)} \tag{16}$$

However, the *perpendicular* mutual compliance, $\alpha_{12}^{\perp}(\omega)$, is calculated with a different proportionality factor (based on perpendicular displacements between probes):

$$G_{12}(\omega) = \frac{1}{8\pi r_{12}\alpha_{12}^{\perp}(\omega)} \left(\frac{\lambda(\omega) + 3G_{12}(\omega)}{\lambda(\omega) + 2G_{12}(\omega)} \right) \tag{17}$$

where the Lamé-coefficients are λ and G (noting that $G = \mu$) and the ratio of the parallel to the perpendicular mutual compliance is 2 at the incompressible limit:

$$\frac{\alpha_{12}^{\|}(\omega)}{\alpha_{12}^{\perp}(\omega)} = 2 \tag{18}$$

Note that here, the radius of the probes are not explicit in the expressions for the mutual complex shear modulus. Instead, the distance between the probes r_{12} is explicit. This implies that with 2-point microrheology, the local effects due to the probe geometry are inconsequential [30].

9 Unfolding Event Counting for Characterizing Biopolymer Unfolding Events

Two-point microrheology is more apt to apply for characterizing single biopolymers directly. Here we derive a novel analysis tool for characterizing unfolding events in

Fig. 2 Microrheology experiment modes. **A**. One particle embedded, passive or active. **B**. Two-point embedded, passive or active. **C**. Two-point linear, passive or active applied on a single fibrous biopolymer. **D**. Two-point linear, passive or active applied on a single globular protein (attached to probes using fibrous biopolymers at either ends). *Arrows* indicate monitored fluctuation axes directions for passive mode; transparent *bi-directional arrow* indicates oscillation direction for active mode

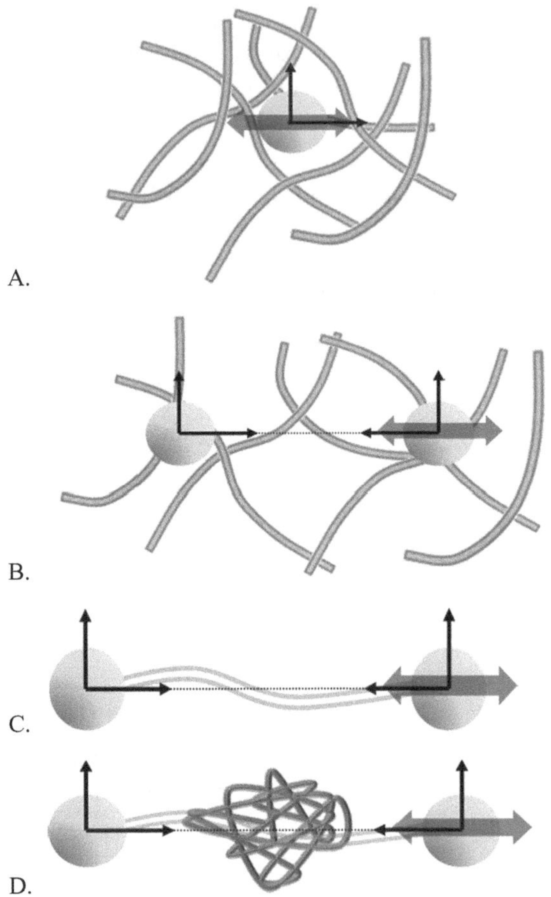

biopolymer of fibrous or globular structures. By attaching a single fibrous biopolymer or a globular protein, between two probes, stretching forces can be applied by moving one of the probes (Fig. 2C and D). The force f applied to move the probe can be implemented at a constant value by slowly increasing the force within a short time τ_o before staying at the constant value (Fig. 3A). We then derive a new approach based on counting unfolding events using the model by Bernido et al., as discussed above [18, 19]. The spectrum of the parallel cross-correlation of the probes is hypothesized to show a dip at the corresponding frequency (*angular frequency ω_o*) of unfolding (Fig. 3B), about the expected spectrum due to thermal fluctuation. The occurrence of the dip would occur due to the anti-correlation between probe fluctuations defined by the following coupled *Langevin equations*:

$$F_1 = -a\sin(\omega t) - ku_1 - \chi\frac{du_1}{dt} + \beta_1(t) \tag{19a}$$

$$F_2 = a\sin(\omega t + \phi) - ku_2 - \chi\frac{du_2}{dt} + \beta_2(t) \tag{19b}$$

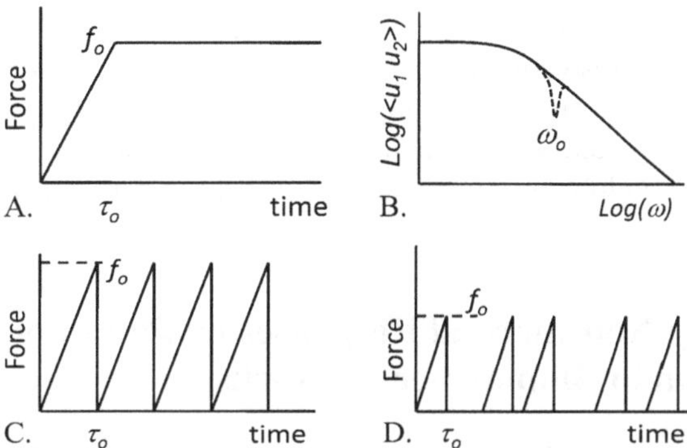

Fig. 3 Stretching experiment modes. **A.** Constant force application. **B.** The dip (at ω_o) in the spectrum due to the anti-correlation of the probes stretching a biopolymer, approximated by the resonance amplitude in a forced damped harmonic oscillator; this characterizes unfolding events in biopolymers under a constant tensile force. **C.** Force pulse train to monitor high frequency response. Amplitude $= f_o$, time constant $= \tau_o$. **D.** Force pulse train with same amplitude and time constant but sequentially randomized

where β_1 and β_2 are uncorrelated thermal noise, ω is the forcing frequency due to unwinding, ϕ, is the phase constant difference between the probe displacements (considered negligible), k, is the effective spring constant (associated with the biopolymer and optical tweezers of identical trapping conditions), with damping coefficient, χ, due to viscous interaction with the solvent, amplitude a of the unwinding. The expected spectral density $C^d(\omega)$ is here approximated to be negatively proportional to the resonance amplitude of a harmonic oscillator with damping coefficient, χ, superposing thermal noise. This amplitude can be directly calculated from the cross-correlation between the stretching probes and would therefore show a dip due to the resonance of the probe fluctuations at opposing displacement directions:

$$C^d(\omega) = \int \langle u_1(t)u_2(t)\rangle \exp(i\omega t)\, dt \tag{20a}$$

$$C^d(\omega) = -A/\left((\omega - \omega_o)^2 + 4\chi_t^2\omega^2\right) + \xi(\omega) \tag{20b}$$

where A is a constant factor, $\xi(\omega)$, is the expected spectrum due to thermal fluctuation and the dip centers at ω_o, which is here interpreted as the natural frequency of the biopolymer (Fig. 3B). The time constant, χ_t, appears due to damping by fluid drag. However the relation of the time constant to the drag coefficient is not expected to be the same relation as in the simple harmonic oscillator with drag. To estimate the number of unfolding events n, we use the time constant, χ_t, and fluctuation resonance, ω_o:

$$n = \frac{\chi_t \omega_o}{2\pi} \tag{21}$$

Provided that the length, L, of the biopolymer is measured while stretching, with unfolding events counted as n, the biopolymer is fully characterized by the winding probability function, $W(n, L)$. The symmetric peaks at the cross-correlations are naturally predicted as resonances due to the mutual harmonic motion of the attached probes reacting to a constant stretching force. A resonance peak corresponds to a winding probability peak, which we now define as descriptive of unfolding events in a biopolymer or a globular protein subjected to a constant tensile force.

10 Simulating Non-thermal Responses by Pulse Force Application in Biopolymer Networks

It follows from the derivations above that measurements of the local and bulk mechanical properties of biopolymer networks are naturally available using one or two-point microrheology (active or passive modes), respectively. Thus, by a comparison of measurements by single or paired probes, one can characterize bulk heterogeneity. And since passive microrheology is based on the assumption that the observed fluctuation is solely due to thermal energy, a comparison with mechanical property measurements using active microrheology, determine non-thermal contributions unaccounted for by FDT [29]. Similarly, non-thermal characterization of biopolymer networks can be done by introducing non-linear strain deformation with controlled force profiles. To do this, a force pulse train of high enough amplitude can be used to deform a single biopolymer or a network configuration (Fig. 3C). Each force pulse simulates accumulative contraction events as observed in biopolymer networks simulating a living cell, which provided a widening of the fluctuation spectra of embedded probes (following a quadratic power law) [31]. This aforementioned study simulated internal contractions in living cells, which are hypothesized to contribute to cellular stiffening. Thus, the pulse train can be further varied by randomizing the occurrence of each pulse in the time series to simulate real force accumulation events within living cells [31–34] (Fig. 3D).

11 Dual-Optical Tweezer Design

We described novel experiment designs above for characterizing unfolding events of fibrous biopolymers and globular proteins by the application of a constant tensile force and a method for simulating randomized force accumulations in biopolymer networks. These approaches are based on the observations of force-displacement curves from embedded (or attached) probe fluctuations and manipulation. The anticipated forces and displacements are at the order of pico-Newtons and nanometers, respectively. An optical tweezer is specifically capable of implementing forces at pN scales and monitoring probe fluctuations at sub-nanometer range using quadrant photodiodes with backfocal plane interferometry [23, 35]. To implement all modes of microrheology described above (active, passive, single particle, or two-point modes, and their combinations), we designed a dual-laser system passing through a differential interference contrast microscope system, with two quadrant

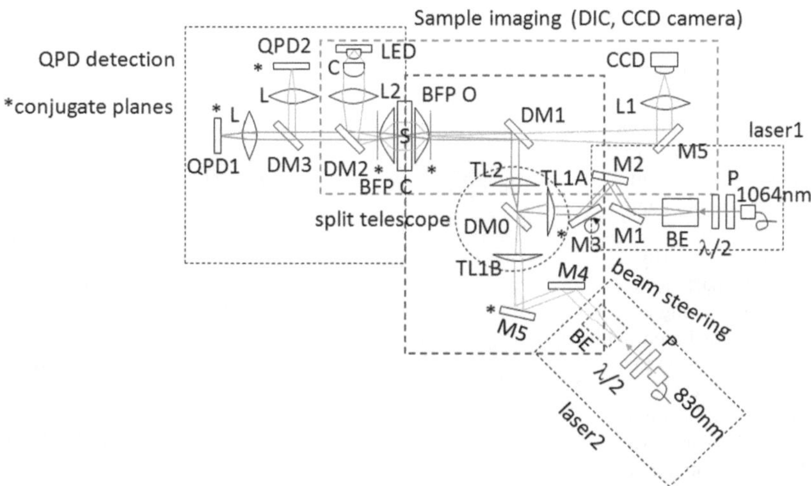

Fig. 4 Optical tweezer system and trapping schemes. Dual optical trap system using 1064 nm and 830 nm lasers. *M*, mirrors; *M3*, steering mirror; *BFP O*, backfocal plane objective; *DM*, dichroic mirror; *TL*, telescope lens; *f*, focal length; *QPD*, quadrant photodiode; *L*, lens; *BFP C*, backfocal plane condenser; *DIC*, differential interference contrast microscopy; *S*, sample; *LED*, light emitting diode; *CCD*, charge-coupled device camera

photodiodes to monitor two probe displacements simultaneously (Fig. 4). Passing through only one microscope objective, the lasers are combined with a "split telescope system" using three lenses in tandem. The manipulating beam is a crystal laser, 700 mW intense, and has a wavelength of 1064 nm, to avoid unnecessary heating of the samples (in water) [36]; but with enough power to trap colloidal particles with radii from hundreds of nm to about 10 micrometers. The monitoring beam is an 830 nm He-Ne low intensity laser. The monitoring beam (830 nm) has a fixed position, whereas the trapping beam (1064 nm) can be steered by using a rotating mirror, which is expected to be mechanically linear until about 100 Hz (beam steering inset, Fig. 4).

12 Discussion and Limitations

One particle microrheology is implemented using this dual-wavelength optical tweezers system by overlapping the trap (1064 nm) and monitoring (830 nm) beams (Fig. 5A). Two-point microrheology is to be performed by separating the beams (Fig. 5B). The optical trap system described here is expected to be optimum in both one particle and two-point microrheology for biopolymer networks or on the surface of bulk materials (e.g., living cells). Active microrheology for either one particle or two-point microrheology is performed with the use of lock-in amplification to monitor displacement responses (measured with the monitoring beam) at the specific frequency of oscillatory mechanical deformation (implemented with the trapping

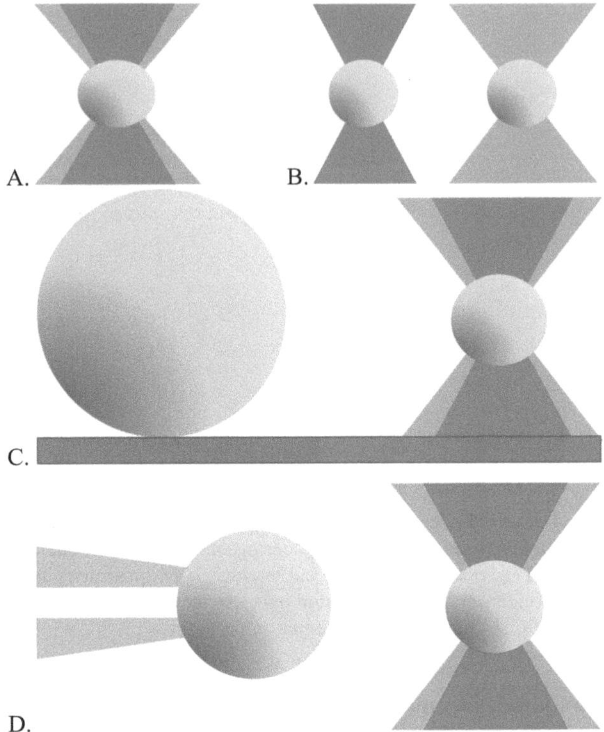

Fig. 5 Beam orientations for optical tweezer experiments. **A**. Overlapping trapping and monitoring beams. **B**. Separate beams. **C**. One particle is immobilized by attachment to the bottom surface with trapping and monitoring beams overlapping on a nearby probe. **D**. One particle is immobilized by using a micropipette attachment with overlapping beams on the other particle. The microrheology of a single fibrous biopolymer or a globular protein attached via biopolymer extensions is possible in **C** and **D**

beam). Note however that the analytical tools developed here to characterize fibrous biopolymers and globular proteins by stretching require that both beams are trapping. However, if one of the attached particles is immobilized either by attachment to the bottom surface (Fig. 5C) or with a micropipette (Fig. 5D), then it is still possible to measure unwinding events by monitoring the auto-correlations of the trapped particle. And we adapt Eqs. (20a), (20b) to instead take the power spectral density $C^s(\omega)$ of the single probe fluctuations (by auto-correlation):

$$C^s(\omega) = \int \langle u(0)u(t) \rangle \exp(i\omega t)\, dt \tag{22a}$$

$$C^s(\omega) = +A/\left((\omega - \omega_o)^2 + (2\chi_t\omega)^2\right) + \xi(\omega) \tag{22b}$$

Here $\xi(\omega)$ is the expected spectral density due to thermal fluctuation superposing the damped harmonic motion amplitude; and the number of unwinding events n is still calculated from the resonance frequency (21). The resonance ω_o is here interpreted as the *natural unwinding frequency* of the fibrous biopolymer or globular protein under a constant tensile force.

However, here we expect instead a peak in the spectral density of the single probe fluctuation, which would be less pronounced. To fully implement the derived analytical tool for counting unwinding events, a more intense 4 W Nd-YAG 1064 nm laser is required. This is to ensure that we have a twin optical trap system strong enough

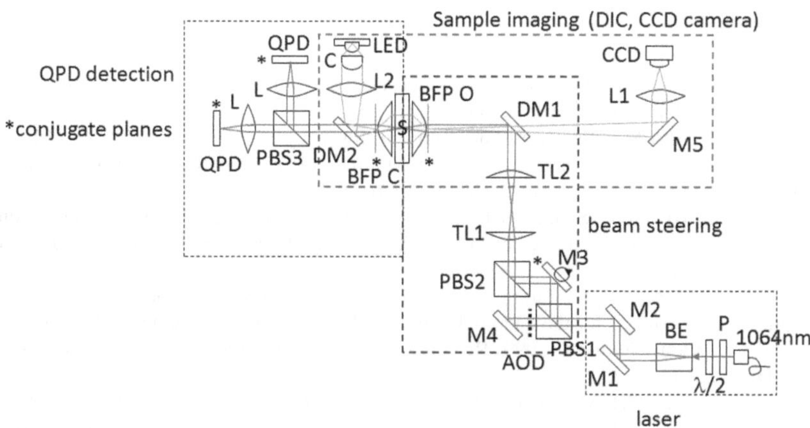

Fig. 6 Twin optical tweezer system. Dual optical trap system using 1064 nm and 830 nm lasers. *AOD*, acousto-optical device; *M*, mirrors; *M3*, steering mirror; *PBS*, polarizing beam splitters; *BFP O*, backfocal plane objective; *DM*, dichroic mirror; *TL*, telescope lens; *f*, focal length; *QPD*, quadrant photodiode; *L*, lens; *BFP C*, backfocal plane condenser; *DIC*, differential interference contrast microscopy; *S*, sample; *CCD*, charge-coupled device camera

for the intended unfolding applications (Fig. 6). The design for the twin optical trap system is based on Moffit et al. (2006), which utilized a rotating mirror with the polarizing beam splitters to separate one laser beam for steering and recombining the steered beam and the other beam before the microscope [37]. However, to approach steering at frequencies above 100 Hz, our novel design inserts an acousto-optical device to steer one of the beams, while the other beam is steered using the rotating mirror, which is capable of linear mechanical steering only within 100 Hz (Fig. 6). Thus, both beams are steered. The limitation however in the use of the same wavelength for trapping and monitoring is the cross-talk at detection (using quadrant photodiodes, QPDs) [24, 38].

The techniques derived in this paper (various microrheology modes and experimental schemes) provide robust tools for characterizing mechanical properties of soft samples that would lead to insights in fundamental biological functions, which are at the forefront for understanding health. However, the applications are further easily extended to soft matter in general, which are not necessarily of biological origin. Furthermore, since the approach is performed at very small volumes (micro-liter range), the benefits are directed specifically where large bulk samples are not available. Results coming from the study of mechanics at microscopic scales surrounding living cells, down to the investigations of unfolding in protein units provide insights on the workings of living matter and therefore opens the avenue for finding novel non-linear and non-equilibrium physical phenomena.

Acknowledgements The research work reported in this paper was partially funded by the University of San Carlos (USC, Cebu City, Philippines) Research Office and the Department of Physics (USC).

References

1. Discher DE, Janmey P, Wang YL (2005) Tissue cells feel and respond to the stiffness of their substrate. Science 310(5751):1139–1143
2. Engler AJ, Griffin MA, Sen S, Bonnemann CG, Sweeney HL, Discher DE (2004) Myotubes differentiate optimally on substrates with tissue-like stiffness: pathological implications for soft or stiff microenvironments. J Cell Biol 166(6):877–887
3. Bacabac RG, Mizuno D, Schmidt CF, MacKintosh FC, Van Loon JJ, Klein-Nulend J, Smit TH (2008) Round versus flat: bone cell morphology, elasticity, and mechanosensing. J Biomech 41(7):1590–1598
4. Nijenhuis N, Mizuno D, Schmidt CF, Vink H, Spaan JA (2008) Microrheology of hyaluronan solutions: implications for the endothelial glycocalyx. Biomacromolecules 9(9):2390–2398
5. Burger EH, Klein-Nulend J (1999) Responses of bone cells to biomechanical forces in vitro. Adv Dent Res 13:93–98
6. Bacabac RG, Smit TH, Mullender MG, Dijcks SJ, Van Loon JJ, Klein-Nulend J (2004) Nitric oxide production by bone cells is fluid shear stress rate dependent. Biochem Biophys Res Commun 315(4):823–829
7. Bacabac RG, Smit TH, Van Loon JJ, Doulabi BZ, Helder M, Klein-Nulend J (2006) Bone cell responses to high-frequency vibration stress: does the nucleus oscillate within the cytoplasm? FASEB J 20(7):858–864
8. Janmey PA, Weitz DA (2004) Dealing with mechanics: mechanisms of force transduction in cells. Trends Biochem Sci 29(7):364–370
9. Endlich N, Otey CA, Kriz W, Endlich K (2007) Movement of stress fibers away from focal adhesions identifies focal adhesions as sites of stress fiber assembly in stationary cells. Cell Motil Cytoskelet 64(12):966–976
10. Gittes F, MacKintosh FC (1998) Dynamic shear modulus of a semiflexible polymer network. Phys Rev E 58(2):R1241
11. Janmey PA, Hvidt S, Kas J, Lerche D, Maggs A, Sackmann E, Schliwa M, Stossel TP (1994) The mechanical properties of actin gels. Elastic modulus and filament motions. J Biol Chem 269(51):32503–32513
12. Storm C, Pastore JJ, MacKintosh FC, Lubensky TC, Janmey PA (2005) Nonlinear elasticity in biological gels. Nature 435(7039):191–194
13. Bendix PM, Koenderink GH, Cuvelier D, Dogic Z, Koeleman BN, Brieher WM, Field CM, Mahadevan L, Weitz DA (2008) A quantitative analysis of contractility in active cytoskeletal protein networks. Biophys J 94(8):3126–3136
14. Piechoka IK, Bacabac RG, Potters M, MacKintosh FC, Koenderink GH (2010) Structural hierarchy governs fibrin gel mechanics. Biophys J 98:2281–2289
15. Alberts B, Johnson A, Lewis J, Raff M, Roberts K, Walter P (2002) Molecular biology of the cell. Garland Science, New York
16. Fung YC (1988) Microrheology and constitutive equation of soft tissue. Biorheology 25(1–2):261–270
17. Smith D, Ziebert F, Humphrey D, Duggan C, Steinbeck M, Zimmermann W, Kas J (2007) Molecular motor-induced instabilities and cross linkers determine biopolymer organization. Biophys J 93(12):4445–4452
18. Bernido CC, Carpio-Bernido MV (2005) Overwinding in a stochastic model of an extended polymer. Phys Lett A 369:1–4
19. Bernido CC, Carpio-Bernido MV, Bornales JB (2005) Overwinding in a stochastic model of an extended polymer. Phys Lett A 339:232–236
20. Crocker JC, Hoffman BD (2007) Multiple-particle tracking and two-point microrheology in cells. Methods Cell Biol 83:141–178
21. Levine AJ, Lubensky TC (2000) One- and two-particle microrheology. Phys Rev Lett 85(8):1774–1777
22. Levine AJ, Lubensky TC (2001) Response function of a sphere in a viscoelastic two-fluid medium. Phys Rev E, Stat Nonlinear Soft Matter Phys 63(4 Pt 1):041510

23. Addas KM, Schmidt CF, Tang JX (2004) Microrheology of solutions of semiflexible biopolymer filaments using laser tweezers interferometry. Phys Rev E, Stat Nonlinear Soft Matter Phys 70(2 Pt 1):021503
24. Atakhorrami M, Addas KM, Schmidt CF (2008) Twin optical traps for two-particle cross-correlation measurements: eliminating cross-talk. Rev Sci Instrum 79(4):043103
25. Janmey PA, Georges PC, Hvidt S (2007) Basic rheology for biologists. Methods Cell Biol 83:3–27
26. Schnurr B, Gittes F, MacKintosh FC, Schmidt CF (1997) Determining microscopic viscoelasticity in flexible and semiflexible polymer networks from thermal fluctuations. Macromolecules 30(25):7781–7792
27. Hegner M, Grange W (2002) Mechanics and imaging of single DNA molecules. J Muscle Res Cell Motil 23(5–6):367–375
28. Baumann CG, Bloomfield VA, Smith SB, Bustamante C, Wang MD, Block SM (2000) Stretching of single collapsed DNA molecules. Biophys J 78(4):1965–1978
29. Mizuno D, Head DA, MacKintosh FC, Schmidt CF (2008) Active and passive microrheology in equilibrium and nonequilibrium systems. Macromolecules 41(19):7194–7202
30. Crocker JC, Valentine MT, Weeks ER, Gisler T, Kaplan PD, Yodh AG, Weitz DA (2000) Two-point microrheology of inhomogeneous soft materials. Phys Rev Lett 85(4):888–891
31. Mizuno D, Tardin C, Schmidt CF, MacKintosh FC (2007) Nonequilibrium mechanics of active cytoskeletal networks. Science 315(5810):370–373
32. Mizuno D, Bacabac RG, Tardin C, Head DA, Schmidt CF (2009) High-resolution probing of cellular force transmission. Phys Rev Lett 102:168102
33. Lau AW, Hoffman BD, Davies A, Crocker JC, Lubensky TC (2003) Microrheology, stress fluctuations, and active behavior of living cells. Phys Rev Lett 91(19):198101
34. MacKintosh FC, Levine AJ (2008) Nonequilibrium mechanics and dynamics of motor-activated gels. Phys Rev Lett 100(1):018104
35. Gittes F, Schmidt CF (1998) Interference model for back-focal-plane displacement detection in optical tweezers. Opt Lett 23(1):7–9
36. Peterman EJ, Gittes F, Schmidt CF (2003) Laser-induced heating in optical traps. Biophys J 84 (2 Pt 1):1308–1316
37. Moffitt JR, Chemla YR, Izhaky D, Bustamante C (2006) Differential detection of dual traps improves the spatial resolution of optical tweezers. Proc Natl Acad Sci USA 103(24):9006–9011
38. Mangeol P, Bockelmann U (2008) Interference and crosstalk in double optical tweezers using a single laser source. Rev Sci Instrum 79(8):083103

Optimization Approaches for the Design of Additively Manufactured Scaffolds

Sara M. Giannitelli, Alberto Rainer, Dino Accoto, Stefano De Porcellinis, Elena M. De-Juan-Pardo, Eugenio Guglielmelli, and Marcella Trombetta

Abstract Scaffolds play a pivotal role in tissue engineering, promoting the synthesis of neo extra-cellular matrix (ECM), and providing temporary mechanical support for the cells during tissue regeneration. Advances introduced by additive manufacturing techniques have significantly improved the ability to regulate scaffold architecture, enhancing the control over scaffold shape and porosity. Thus, considerable research efforts have been devoted to the fabrication of 3D porous scaffolds with optimized micro-architectural features. This chapter gives an overview of the methods for the design of additively manufactured scaffolds and their applicability in tissue engineering (TE). Along with a survey of the state of the art, the Authors will also present a recently developed method, called Load-Adaptive Scaffold Architecturing (LASA), which returns scaffold architectures optimized for given applied mechanical loads systems, once the specific stress distribution is evaluated through Finite Element Analysis (FEA).

1 Introduction

Scaffolds are central to tissue engineering (TE), as they provide a suitable environment for cell adhesion, proliferation, and production of neo-extracellular matrix (ECM), while ensuring a temporary mechanical support during tissue regeneration.

S.M. Giannitelli · A. Rainer · M. Trombetta
Tissue Engineering Laboratory, CIR-Center for Integrated Research, Università Campus
Bio-Medico di Roma, via Alvaro del Portillo 21, 00128 Rome, Italy

D. Accoto · E. Guglielmelli
Biomedical Robotics and Biomicrosystems Laboratory, CIR-Center for Integrated Research,
Università Campus Bio-Medico di Roma, via Alvaro del Portillo 21, 00128 Rome, Italy

S. De Porcellinis
Biomatica Srl, via G. Peroni 442/444, 00131 Rome, Italy

E.M. De-Juan-Pardo
Tissue Engineering and Biomaterials Unit, CEIT and Tecnun, University of Navarra, Manuel de
Lardizábal 15, 20018 San Sebastián, Spain

P.R. Fernandes, P.J. Bártolo (eds.), *Tissue Engineering*,
Computational Methods in Applied Sciences 31, DOI 10.1007/978-94-007-7073-7_6,
© Springer Science+Business Media Dordrecht 2014

In the last decade, technologies for the preparation of biomaterial scaffolds benefited from the development of several additive manufacturing (AM) techniques, which allowed the production of free-form porous scaffolds with custom-tailored architectures that can be easily derived from solid models obtained, for example, from diagnostic medical imaging. Among the AM techniques most commonly used in TE, we can include: selective laser sintering (SLS), stereolithography (SLA), extrusion-based techniques (e.g. fused deposition modeling, precision extrusion deposition) and three dimensional printing (3DP) [1]. These techniques have been widely investigated for the processing of thermoplastic biopolymers into structures with controlled shape and tailored porosity and have been successfully applied for the preparation of several scaffolds for different applications, such as bone TE [2, 3] repair of osteochondral defects [4–6], and lumbar interbody fusion implants [7].

Advances introduced by AM techniques have significantly improved the ability to control scaffold architecture (size, shape, interconnectivity, geometry, and orientation), yielding to biomimetic structures with different design and material compositions, thereby enhancing control over their mechanical properties, biological effects, and degradation kinetics. Integration of AM with medical imaging techniques has allowed the production of scaffolds that are customized in size and shape for specific applications or even for individual patients.

The use of computer-based technologies in TE has quickly evolved into the development of a new field, named Computer-Aided Tissue Engineering (CATE). It can be defined as the application of enabling computer-aided technologies, including computer-aided design (CAD), image processing, computer-aided manufacturing (CAM), and rapid prototyping (RP) for modeling, designing, simulating, and manufacturing biological tissue and organ substitutes. Taking advantage from these tools, scaffold design, intended as the selection of material and micro-architecture proper for a specific application, has gained growing interest within TE. The central role of scaffold microstructure in determining the functionality of both the construct and the newly grown tissue, has been clearly demonstrated [8, 9]. Thus, research efforts are moving towards the development of innovative methods for the generation of scaffold architectures optimized on the basis of application-specific biological and mechanical requirements. In this context, Finite Element Analysis (FEA) has played a main role in the reduction of experimental tests and costs required by *in vitro* and *in vivo* research.

The present chapter gives an overview of the methods for the design of additively manufactured scaffolds and their applicability in TE. Along with a survey of the state of the art, the Authors will also present a recently developed method, called *load-adaptive scaffold architecturing (LASA)*, which is based on the finite element calculation of the stress field at the scaffold site on the basis of an imposed load system.

2 Scaffold Design and Optimization

Several approaches have been described in the literature for the design of scaffolds with subject-specific external shapes along with controlled internal microarchitectures. Most of these studies rely on the use of unit cells with well-known geometric, mechanical, and fluid-flow properties, which can be assembled together according to the application needs. Boolean operations between the 3D reconstruction of the defect site and the arranged stack of cellular units are required for the construction of the final design. Hence, different libraries of unit cells have been created, and algorithms have been developed to allow their automatic design and assembly [10]. CAD-based libraries have been developed starting from regular polyhedral shapes [11, 12] or using Boolean intersections between a solid domain and geometric primitives, such as spheres and cylinders, to create the void spaces of the porous element [12]. More recently, the use of unit cells based on CAD representation of triply periodic minimal surfaces (e.g. gyroid and diamond) has been proposed [13, 14]. When replicated and assembled at the macro scale, these morphologies showed a positive influence on cell migration and tissue in-growth while representing an optimal biomorphic tissue architecture [15]. Furthermore, an image-based approach has been introduced by Hollister et al. to design scaffold unit cells simply setting voxels within a representative design element to 0 or 1, depending on the presence or the absence of the material in the corresponding region. Several strategies have been adopted for the creation of a variety of topologies with both regular and randomly distributed pores within the unit cell [16]. Image-based designs, fitting diagnostic imaging data, have been generated and successively coupled with optimization algorithms to match existing host tissue mechanical properties [17].

Another particular cellular solid has been obtained by stacking alternate layers of filaments, such as those fabricated via extrusion-based AM techniques, according to selected patterns. The use of these processing techniques required the introduction of specific computer-aided tools in order to obtain the desired material distribution profile in a continuous and interconnected way throughout the entire geometry. Varying architectural parameters such as fiber diameter, spacing between consecutive fibers, layer thickness and deposition angle between layers, 3D scaffolds with controlled porosity, pore shape and tailored mechanical properties have been obtained [18–20]. In a recent study, Sobral et al. demonstrated how additive manufacturing techniques are suitable at modifying architectural features of the scaffold with the aim of increasing mechanical stability and cell seeding efficacy [21]. Space-filling fractal curves, such as Hilbert curves, have been also used in combination with extrusion-based methods for the generation of internal architectures mimicking bone gradient porosity [22].

Even if the use of regular lattice structures has lead to several advantages in terms of modeling, fabrication, properties evaluation and prediction, they are not suited to fully represent the complexity of heterogeneous natural tissues. To this aim, efforts have been made in order to create more intricate internal architectures and/or to find irregular ways to assemble the elemental cells. Thus, libraries of more complex units have been fabricated while new packing approaches have been developed in order to generate stochastically the anchors points of each unit element [23, 24].

A totally different approach to obtain more realistic 3D models is based on the reconstruction of the tissue (e.g. bone) morphology, starting from computer tomography (CT) or other digital imaging data [25–27]. However, designing a faithful copy of real structures is difficult, time consuming and in most cases not strictly necessary; therefore, capturing and reproducing the main key properties of natural structures (such as porosity and pore distribution) in an effective yet simple manner could represent a valid alternative to obtain the desired results [28, 29].

For years, a 'trial-and-error' approach has been adopted to validate scaffold micro-architectures, with modifications being made to an existing design on the basis of *in vitro* or *in vivo* results [30]. More recently, Finite Element Analysis (FEA) contributed to the reduction of experimental tests and to shortening scaffold design process. FEA has been at first used in TE for a *post hoc* investigation of the mechanical behavior of scaffolds and to predict their interactions with the surrounding tissues. For example, several finite element studies provided a computational approach to evaluate the effects of mechanical stimuli induced by fluid flow and mechanical loads to the cells seeded into a scaffold [31, 32]; the computed results were used to modify geometrical or material parameters and to choose the most suitable ones for tissue replacement. CAD and μCT-based models of the produced porous scaffolds have been normally considered as input geometry. The reasonable accuracy of simulation results, in comparison with experimental data, has led to the recent use of FEA as a predictive tool for the *a priori* design and optimization of scaffold architectures [33].

When approaching the fabrication of porous scaffolds, two main issues have to be simultaneously addressed: one is the optimal porosity, which will depend on the ability of hosted cells to migrate and proliferate within the scaffold; the other one regards the capability of the produced scaffold to bear physiological loads once implanted, without dramatic collapses [34]. The latter issue is particularly urging in the case of scaffolds intended for the regeneration of mineralized tissue, where the scaffold implant should provide a leading framework for the repair of the damage. The need for an optimization problem therefore emerges: on the one hand, the ideal scaffold should exhibit a sufficiently large porosity; on the other hand, it should be stiff and robust enough to withstand physiological loads. Such requirements are evidently antagonistic, since a large porosity negatively impacts robustness. For this reason, the development of design strategies capable to optimal trade-off between these two opposite needs is one of the main challenges of TE.

Topological optimization techniques are often used in combination with FEA in order to obtain functional scaffold microarchitectures that maximize stiffness while preserving constraints on the total mass budget. They aim at achieving the best use of material within a structure subjected to either a single load or a multiple load distribution and involve the determination of features such as location, number and shape of "holes", as well as connectivity of the domain, in order to compute new microstructures that attain desired properties [35]. Thus, instead of relying on CAD tools to design unit cell geometries, topology optimization approaches have been used to locate void and solid spaces within the initial domain on the basis of the desired tissue requirements. A pioneering work in this context is represented by the study of Almeida et al. [36], who developed a tool combining CAD-based modeling and analytic methods to simulate and optimize scaffolds providing an *a priori* control of the mechanical properties as a function of porosity and scaffold architecture. Instead of starting form a predefined unit cell, the tool starts form a dense non-porous block of material, searching for a topologically optimized scaffold unit according to porosity and stiffness requirements.

Following the success of topology optimization methods, both the number of parameters implemented during FEA analysis as well as the conditions studied in a real representation of physical environment, have increased tremendously. As an example, mechano-regulation models have been recently developed to study the biophysical stimulus exerted by different scaffold microstructures on the cells and hence their effect on the regenerative process [37–39]. Results derived from these studies pointed out the considerable impact of scaffold micro-architecture on tissue regeneration outcome and contributed to the development of hugely optimized designs.

2.1 Topological Optimization by Load-Adaptive Scaffold Architecturing (LASA) Algorithm

The present method envisages an innovative strategy for the fabrication of highly optimized structures, based on an *a priori* FEA of the physiological load set at the implant site. The resulting scaffold micro-architecture does not follow a regular geometrical pattern; on the contrary, it is based on the results of a numerical study. The algorithm was applied to a solid free-form fabrication process, using poly(ε-caprolactone) (PCL) as the starting material for the processing of additive manufactured structures. The proposed methodology is initially presented for a simple proof-of-principle geometry and then extended to an illustrative case study, considering a 3D model of the proximal femur, subject to physiological loading conditions. Femur bone was chosen as a target, since it represents an anatomic part with well described biomechanical behavior.

2.1.1 Theory and Calculation

Given an elastic continuum $\mathbf{C}$, to which a load system is applied, the stress at every point P of the domain is described by a stress tensor σ ($\in \mathbb{R}^{3\times3}$). Being σ symmetrical for reasons of statics, for every P there exists an orthonormal reference frame $\mathbf{R}$, which makes σ diagonal. The three components of the diagonalized stress tensor, σ_1, σ_2, and σ_3 are the so-called principal stresses, which correspond to pure compression/tension occurring along the three axes (x_1, x_2, x_3) of $\mathbf{R}$. A technique for ideally carving within $\mathbf{C}$, while minimizing the reduction of stiffness, consists in placing the residual material along the principal directions, thus minimizing the distortion of the structure due to shear stresses.

With this consideration, the best solution for the definition of the scaffold design could be to drive the position and direction of the solid material according to the vector field of the principal stresses. Being the *trabeculae* oriented along principal stress directions, they work in almost pure tension/compression mode, which results

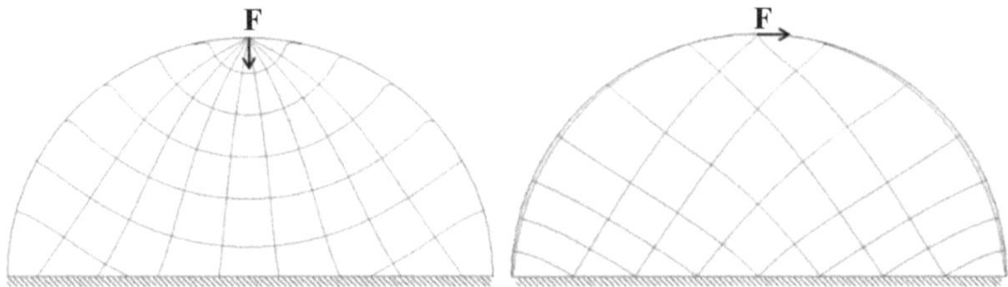

Fig. 1 Plot of the principal stress directions (σ_1 and σ_2) for two different loading conditions

in higher stiffness. Structures fabricated following these criteria were conceived to obtain a lightweight material distribution as early as in the 1900s [40] and have been found to represent the optimized solution chosen by the nature to arrange the material in most skeletal bones [41]. Thus, the goal of an optimal implant should be to keep the stress distribution after its insertion close to the physiological stress distribution. With this intent, several physiological models devoted to visualize these distribution profiles have been developed, especially in case of femur bone [42].

In particular, principal stresses vector field can be numerically evaluated using FEA, and the corresponding principal stress lines can be post-processed in a suitable environment to obtain the toolpath for an additive manufacturing system. A direct control of scaffold porosity and pore distribution is achievable by simply regulating the spacing (and consequently the number) of the trabecular structures. A strategy to obtain principal stress lines equally distributed throughout the entire design domain consists in choosing seeding points uniformly spaced along the design space boundary. Alternatively, a new sampling curve could be specifically introduced in to design domain; in both cases, curves sampling will generate the starting points of the trabecular elements. Furthermore, a different selection of principal stress lines could also be adopted in order to manufacture scaffolds with required gradient porosity.

For the validation of the proposed approach, a simple geometry for the domain **C** was considered. The geometry consisted of a semicircle, with a radius of 2 cm, clamped at the bottom along its diameter, and loaded with a 10 N force applied on the top, being either perpendicular (compressive load) or parallel to the above-mentioned diameter (shear load). The FEA problem was solved using COMSOL Multiphysics (COMSOL, Inc., Burlington, MA), in the hypothesis of plane stress. On the basis of the linear elasticity theory, for an isotropic material within the range of elastic deformation, the direction of the principal stress is neither related to load intensity, nor to the material elastic constants. As both this features do not affect optimal topology, the final design of the scaffold will be exactly the same in case of domains with different load values and material properties. Moreover, position and direction of applied load as well as types of constraints should strongly affect principal stress field. As example, Fig. 1 reports streamlines for principal stresses (σ_1 and σ_2) for the two different loading conditions.

From these considerations we can assess that the resulting micro-architecture design is therefore both geometry-specific (valid for the assigned design domain) and load-specific, while it is not influenced by the material used in fabrication process.

2.1.2 Design and Finite Element Simulations

LASA architecture can be derived from the solution of the above described problem and used to predict and/or optimize scaffold mechanical performance. The geometry of the reticular structure can be obtained orienting the trabecular elements as the envelope of the first and third principal stress directions, with seed points regularly spaced along the diameter in order to obtain a desired total porosity. Thickness of the trabecular elements should be set according both to the resolution of the additive manufacturing fabrication technique and to the printing parameters.

FE evaluation of the mechanical properties of the LASA pattern was performed and compared to that of a control architecture. 2D models of both scaffold architectures were reproduced using a CAD software (AutoCad, Autodesk, San Rafael, CA). The LASA geometry was obtained as above described, choosing seed points regularly spaced along the diameter (Fig. 2a). As a control, a second architecture (rectangular grid, GRID) was designed with linear struts alternatively oriented at $0°$ and $90°$, to create a trabecular structure (Fig. 2b). This architecture was chosen because of its common use for additively manufactured scaffolds. Thickness of the trabecular elements was set at 400 μm, while their number and spacing were arranged to keep the total porosity—i.e. the ratio between the area of the *trabeculae* and the total area of the semicircular domain—constant for the two models (61 % porosity).

CAD geometries were then imported into COMSOL Structural Mechanics Module with the above described compressive load and boundary conditions. The elastic problem was solved and von Mises stress and elastic strain energy density evaluated. Materials properties were selected for PCL ($E = 230$ MPa, Poisson's ratio $v = 0.35$, as experimentally derived from tensile tests on PCL extruded filaments), and a thickness of 1 mm was associated to the 2D model for calculation purposes.

Solution data were exported in terms of nodes, elements and values matrices, and imported into MATLAB (The MathWorks Inc., Natick, MA) for further post-processing. Area-weighted mean stress was calculated according to:

$$\sigma_{vM}^* = \frac{\sum_i (\sigma_{vM})_i \cdot w_i}{\sum_i w_i} \tag{1}$$

where $(\sigma_{vM})_i$ is the value of von Mises stress for the ith element, w_i is the area of the ith element, and $\sum_i w_i$ is the total area of the mesh domain. Stiffness k [N/m] was calculated starting from the following equations:

$$F = k\delta$$
$$U_e = \frac{1}{2}k\delta^2 \tag{2}$$

Hence:

$$k = \frac{F^2}{2U_e} \tag{3}$$

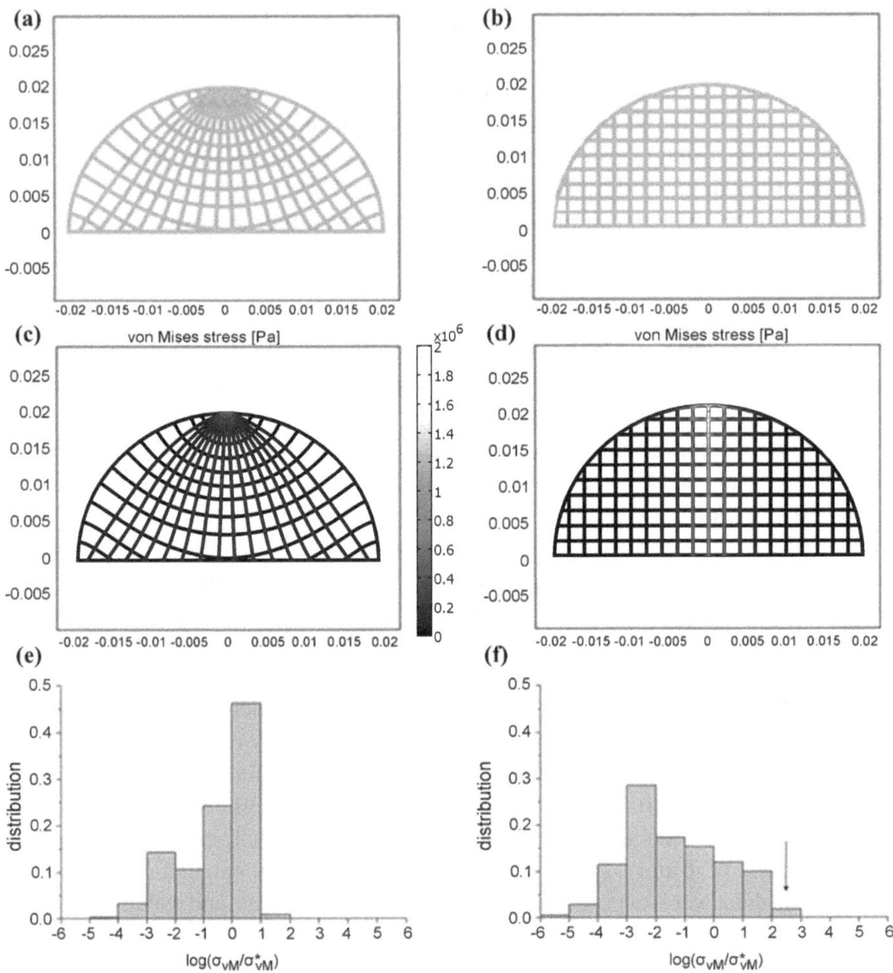

Fig. 2 CAD geometries of the different design rules applied to the semicircular geometry: LASA pattern (**a**) and GRID pattern (**b**). Von Mises stress distribution for LASA (**c**) and GRID (**d**) design. Ratio between local von Mises stress value (σ_{vM}) and mean stress value (σ_{vM}^{*}): distribution histograms for LASA (**e**) and GRID (**f**) (adapted from [43])

where F [N] is the imposed load, δ [m] is the displacement and U_e [J] is the elastic strain energy, calculated as the integral of the strain energy density u [J/m^2] over the domain:

$$U_e = \int_S u \, dS \tag{4}$$

Figure 2 shows the results of FEA on the 2D CAD models obtained by the implementation of the two different design rules—LASA and GRID—applied to the simple benchmark geometry. Although the two models presented almost identical

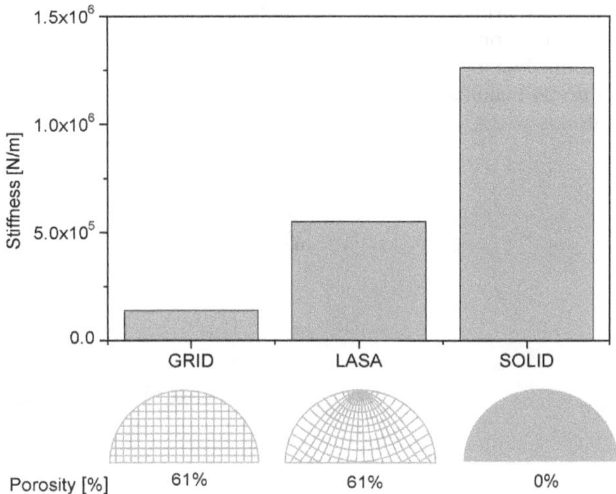

Fig. 3 Stiffness values for LASA and GRID architectures. The stiffness of solid body is also presented as a reference

surface area, corresponding to a porosity of 61 %, they showed different behavior in terms of load bearing.

As it can be observed by the plots (Figs. 2c and 2d) representing the magnitude of von Mises stress over all the elements, the maximum stress value is lower for LASA model. Additionally, mean stress was found to be lower for LASA architecture with respect to GRID architecture (1.02 vs. 1.21 MPa). For the sake of clarity, the same scale was used in Figs. 2c and 2d. In order to exclude singularities, a circular portion of the geometry (1 mm radius) centered on the point of application of the concentrated load, was omitted from representation.

Further analysis on stress distribution showed that it is peaked around the mean value for the LASA model (Fig. 2e). In the GRID model, on the contrary, most of the structure is stressed at values two to three orders of magnitude lower than the mean stress, with a small portion of the structure being highly stressed (Fig. 2f).

Stiffness values are compared in Fig. 3. In addition, data for a solid PCL body with outer dimensions corresponding to the continuum **C** (SOLID model) were added for comparison reasons. It can be observed how LASA architecture presented a higher stiffness with respect to GRID model. Interestingly, its value had the same order of magnitude of the solid model ($k_{LASA}/k_{SOLID} \approx 0.44$), despite its porosity of over 60 %.

Mechanical properties of additively manufactured structures reproduced according to LASA and GRID models were also empirically evaluated under loading conditions similar to those used for FEA. Solids were fabricated using PCL (Mn = 80,000 g/mol, Sigma, Milwaukee, WI), using an AM equipment developed by the authors. The apparatus comprises an AISI 316L stainless steel heated dispensing head with a 21G nozzle at the end, an X–Y motorized stage assembled from two cross-mounted linear stages (model PLS-85 miCos GmbH, Eschbach, Germany) for the positioning of the dispensing head, and a Z-axis (PLS-85, miCos) for controlling its distance from the stage. The motorized stages are connected to a computer

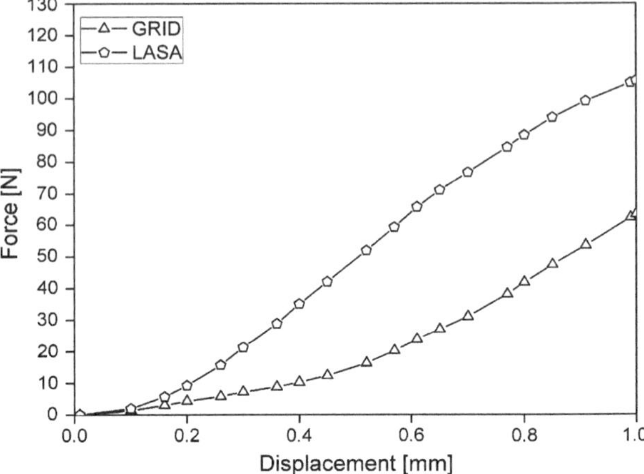

Fig. 4 Experimental results of compression test performed on the PCL additively manufactured scaffolds

programmable motion controller (model SM-32, miCos) and powered by a dedicated power amplifier (model MPA, miCos). The dispensing head is embedded into an aluminum heating mantle, consisting of two heating cartridges and a resistance thermometer (Pt100), connected to a programmable temperature controller (model 400, Gefran, Brescia, Italy). Dispensing is pressure-assisted, and is performed by pressurizing the extrusion head with argon gas by means of a control electrovalve. A custom-developed control software generates the process toolpath and controls the actuation of all the system components. Temperature of the extrusion head was set to 85 °C, and relative speed between the nozzle and the X–Y table was set to 5 mm/s. A total of eight layers were deposited for each scaffold.

Performances of LASA and GRID architectures were evaluated by means of mechanical testing in deformation-controlled mode. Scaffolds were clamped along the diameter to a rigid aluminum plate, positioned on the basement of a mechanical test machine (model 3365, Instron, Norwood, MA), equipped with a 500 N load cell. Samples were loaded on top with a 10 mm diameter cylindrical puncher at a deformation rate of 1 mm/min, until a displacement of 1 mm was reached. Figure 4 shows the resulting force-displacement curve. For every displacement, the load on the LASA structure was higher than on the GRID structure. This is in close agreement with the simulation results, confirming that LASA architecture presented a higher stiffness to compressive loading with respect to the GRID one. These results demonstrate how design rules chosen for the fabrication of additively manufactured scaffolds truly affected the mechanical properties of produced implants and, at the same time, how the LASA architecture is effective in providing a more uniform stress distribution over the trabecular elements.

From a different point of view, a finite element study can be also implemented before scaffold fabrication with the aim to analyze the influence of extrusion parameters on scaffold mechanical performance and choose the most suitable ones for the specific application. Starting from calculated principal stress directions, different patterns can be generated by simply varying the distance between the streamlines and/or the fiber thickness. Such architectures lead to different stiffness values,

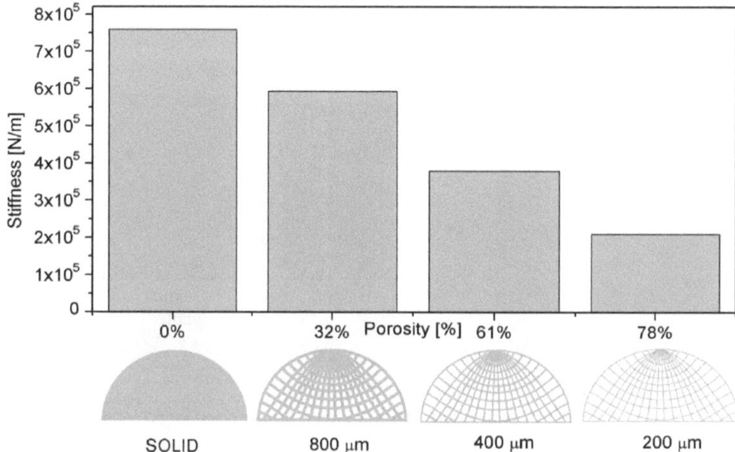

Fig. 5 Stiffness values for structures obtained according to a given LASA pattern as a function of porosity. The stiffness of solid body is presented as a reference

in combination with different porosity levels and pores dimensions. Thus, starting from a given LASA solution, an optimization process can be carried out, modifying design parameters until a good compromise among trabecular diameter (constrained by the additive manufacture equipment), scaffold porosity and stiffness (related to the specific tissue application), has been reached.

Three different LASA structures with different porosity (78 %, 61 % and 32 %) were generated keeping constant the number and spacing of the trabecular elements, while setting the thickness to 200, 400 and 800 μm, respectively. 2D CAD geometries were imported in COMSOL and stiffness was calculated according to Eq. (3). Figure 5 shows the different stiffness achieved by these geometries. A solid model with dimensions corresponding to the continuum C has been added for comparison reasons. As expected, stiffness increases with increasing fibers thickness approaching the value assumed by the continuum solid geometry.

As an additional simulation, LASA structures were generated with different trabecular thickness (200, 400 and 800 μm), but keeping constant the total porosity value, by changing number and spacing of the fibers. In these conditions, although the cross section of each *trabecula* was increased, the reduction in the number of load-bearing elements resulted in an overall decrease of stiffness values (Fig. 6).

Taken together, these considerations suggest that the proposed LASA approach could provide a useful tool in designing tissue scaffolds with tailored morphology and mechanical behavior.

2.1.3 Model Application

In view of a possible application to the fabrication of scaffolds for TE, the proposed technique has been evaluated on a clinically relevant anatomic portion.

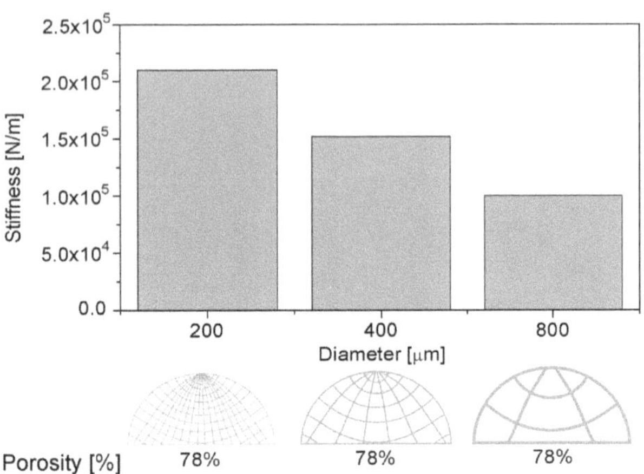

Fig. 6 Stiffness values for structures with the same total porosity obtained according to different scaffold architectures achieved by increasing fiber spacing and thickness

The femur head was chosen, subject to physiological loading conditions. In principle, using clinical CT scans and extracting the region of interest (ROI) with a commercial software (e.g., Mimics, Materialise NV, Leuven, Belgium), subject-specific geometries can be processed. For the purposes of the present study, however, a widely accepted 3D model of an adult human femur was used (3rd generation composite femur, Dept. Mechanical and Industrial Engineering, Ryerson University, Ontario, Canada) [44]. The model was further simplified by considering the whole femur as constituted by an isotropic linear elastic material with homogeneous Young's modulus and constant Poisson's ratio. Although bone is actually heterogeneous, non-linear and anisotropic, these simplifications are often made when modeling bone using FEA [45, 46]. The femur bone domain was discretized by 19,079 tetrahedral 4-nodes elements. Previous studies have confirmed that tetrahedron is the best choice for meshing human femur and that it is well suited to model irregular geometries, due to its quadratic displacement behavior [47].

For the purposes of the present study, a force of 250 N parallel to the femur shaft axis was applied on the top surface of the femur head, distributed on a circular area of 1.5 cm radius. In the pioneering work by Koch [48], describing the laws of bone architecture—following the early studies by Wolff and Cullman—load on the femur was assumed approximately 30 % of the body weight in the bilateral standing position. The line of action of the force was defined as the line joining the center of the head of the femur to the center of gravity of the lower end of this bone. Further studies have demonstrated the importance of taking into account forces exerted by muscles on the femur head, especially for describing single-limb stand [49]. However, simplified loading conditions have often been used, such as concentrated loads directed along the femur shaft direction [50] or, alternatively, at an angle of 20° to the shaft axis in the coronal plane [51].

The FE problem was solved in COMSOL Multiphysics under the hypothesis of static linear analysis. Pointwise stress tensor and principal stress directions were calculated for the entire femur volume. A text file containing the directions of principal stresses as a function of the position was generated and exported into MAT-

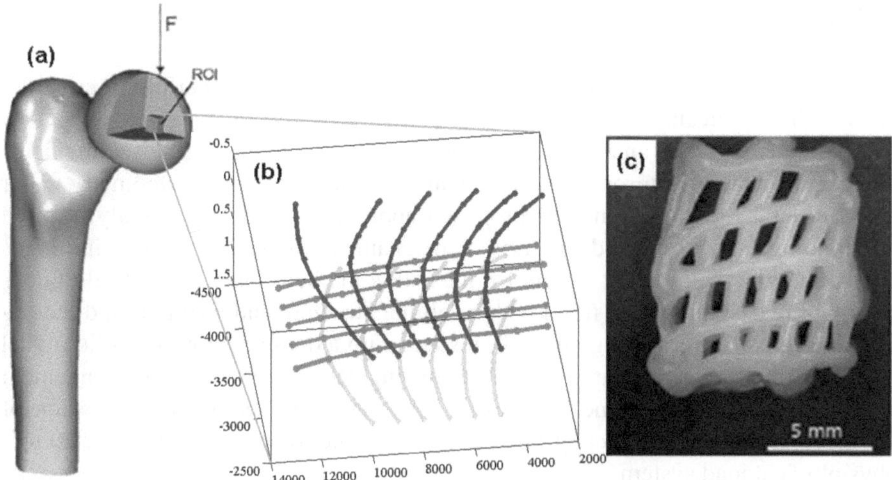

Fig. 7 (**a**) Loading scheme considered for the application of LASA. A portion of the femur head has been removed in the figure to visualize the ROI. (**b**) Calculation of the envelope curves defining the trabecular elements of the LASA architecture. *Curves* indicate the projection of two principal stress directions on the XY-plane for the first three printing layers. (**c**) PCL scaffold obtained by additive manufacturing according to the calculated LASA pattern (adapted from [43])

LAB. Curves following the principal stress directions were traced and further post processing was necessary to automatically generate control primitives compatible to standard CAM language. However, only data relative to a specific ROI were post-processed and visualized.

A small cubic volume within the femur head was selected for the scaffold fabrication (Fig. 7a). In particular, the orientation was chosen so that its faces were aligned to standard anatomical planes. With reference to conventional nomenclature, the printing process occurred on a coronal plane (*i.e.* the coronal plane represents the printer XY plane). A slicing distance of 500 μm was used for the definition of the deposition layers. For each layer, the projections—on the coronal plane—of two principal stress directions were calculated using MATLAB and used for the determination of envelope curves for the ROI. Care was taken in selecting the seed point of each principal stress trajectory in order to achieve the specified distance between trabecular structures. The result of this process was a series of equally spaced 2D plots, corresponding to different cross-sections, each at a slightly different Z-coordinate value. Figure 7b shows a detail of the plot trajectories for the first 3 deposition layers, which are obtained as envelops of the projections of two principal stress directions on the coronal plane.

The obtained slices were used to design and manufacture a small scaffold fitting a portion of the femur head. MATLAB routines were developed to convert such plots into control primitives for the scaffold fabrication. Scaffolds were printed in PCL with the above described additive manufacturing equipment. The resulting PCL structure is represented in Fig. 7c.

3 Conclusions

Topological optimization holds promise to design engineered scaffold microstructures for TE applications.

This study proposes an approach for successfully designing scaffolds with microarchitecture predicted through *a priori* analysis of the implant site geometry under a physiological load system. The proposed approach is both biologically inspired and topologically optimized in terms of mechanical properties, for specific loads and boundary conditions. It differs from existing methods because, instead of considering the design domain filled with a cellular structure and trying to find the optimal design of the repeating unit cell, it starts with a dense continuous solid model and finds the best trabecular architecture, by engineering the material arrangement within the considered volume. The design domain is identified by the outer shape of the defect and the mechanical properties of the tissue to be replaced subjected to a physiological load system.

References

1. Bártolo PJS, Almeida H, Laoui T (2009) Rapid prototyping and manufacturing for tissue engineering scaffolds. Int J Comput Appl Technol 36:1–9
2. Williams JM, Adewunmi A, Schek RM, Flanagan CL, Krebsbacha PH, Feinberg SE, Hollister SJ, Das S (2005) Bone tissue engineering using polycaprolactone scaffolds fabricated via selective laser sintering. Biomaterials 26:4817–4827
3. Simpson RL, Wiria FE, Amis AA, Chua CK, Leong KF, Hansen UN, Chandrasekaran M, Lee MW (2008) Development of a 95/5 poly(L-lactide-co-glycolide)/hydroxylapatite and β-tricalcium phosphate scaffold as bone replacement material via selective laser sintering. J Biomed Mater Res, Part B, Appl Biomater 84B:17–25. doi:10.1002/jbm.b.30839
4. Swieszkowski W, Tuan BHS, Kurzydlowski KJ, Hutmacher DW (2007) Repair and regeneration of osteochondral defects in the articular joints. Biomol Eng 24:489–495
5. Lee CH, Cook JL, Mendelson A, Moioli EK, Yao H, Mao JJ (2010) Regeneration of the articular surface of the rabbit synovial joint by cell homing: a proof of concept study. Lancet 376:440–448
6. Shao X, Goh JC, Hutmacher DW, Lee EH, Zigang G (2006) Repair of large articular osteochondral defects using hybrid scaffolds and bone marrow-derived mesenchymal stem cells in a rabbit model. Tissue Eng 12:1539–1551
7. Abbah SA, Lam CX, Hutmacher DW, Goh JC, Wong HK (2009) Biological performance of a polycaprolactone-based scaffold used as fusion cage device in a large animal model of spinal reconstructive surgery. Biomaterials 30:5086–5093
8. Melchels FPW, Barradas AMC, van Blitterswijk CA, de Boer J, Feijen J, Grijpma DW (2010) Effects of the architecture of tissue engineering scaffolds on cell seeding and culturing. Acta Biomater 6:4208–4217
9. Sanz-Herrera JA, Garcìa-Aznar JM, Doblare M (2009) On scaffold designing for bone regeneration: a computational multiscale approach. Acta Biomater 5:219–229
10. Cheah CM, Chua CK, Leong KF, Cheong CH, Naing MW (2004) Automatic algorithm for generating complex polyhedral scaffolds for tissue engineering. Tissue Eng 10:595–610
11. Chua CK, Leong KF, Cheah CM, Chua SW (2003) Development of a tissue engineering scaffold structure library for rapid prototyping. Part 1: Investigation and classification. Int J Adv Manuf Technol 21:291–301. doi:10.1007/s001700300034

12. Wettergreen MA, Bucklen BS, Starly B, Yuksel E, Sun W, Liebschner MAK (2005) Creation of a unit block library of architectures for use in assembled scaffold engineering. Comput Aided Des 37:1141–1149

13. Rajagopalan S, Robb RA (2006) Schwarz meets Schwann: design and fabrication of biomorphic and durataxic tissue engineering scaffolds. Med Image Anal 10:693–712. doi:10.1016/j.media.2006.06.001

14. Dong JY (2011) Porous scaffold design using the distance field and triply periodic minimal surface models. Biomaterials 32:7741–7754. doi:10.1016/j.biomaterials.2011.07.019

15. Melchels FPW, Bertoldi K, Gabbrielli R, Velders AH, Feijen J, Grijpma DW (2010) Mathematically defined tissue engineering scaffold architectures prepared by stereolithography. Biomaterials 31:6909–6916

16. Hollister SJ, Levy RA, Chu T-M, Halloran JW, Feinberg SE (2000) An image-based approach for designing and manufacturing craniofacial scaffolds. Int J Oral Maxillofac Surg 29:67–71. doi:10.1016/s0901-5027(00)80128-9

17. Hollister SJ (2005) Porous scaffold design for tissue engineering. Nat Mater 4:518–524

18. Woodfield TBF, Malda J, de Wijn J, Péters F, Riesle J, van Blitterswijk CA (2004) Design of porous scaffolds for cartilage tissue engineering using a three-dimensional fiber-deposition technique. Biomaterials 25:4149–4161. doi:10.1016/j.biomaterials.2003.10.056

19. Hutmacher DW, Schantz T, Zein I, Ng KW, Teoh SH, Tan KC (2001) Mechanical properties and cell cultural response of polycaprolactone scaffolds designed and fabricated via fused deposition modeling. J Biomed Mater Res 55:203–216

20. Woodfield TBF, Moroni L, Malda J (2009) Combinatorial approaches to controlling cell behaviour and tissue formation in 3D via rapid-prototyping and smart scaffold design. Comb Chem High Throughput Screen 12:562–579. doi:10.2174/138620709788681899

21. Sobral JM, Caridade SG, Sousa RA, Mano JF, Reis RL (2011) Three-dimensional plotted scaffolds with controlled pore size gradients: effect of scaffold geometry on mechanical performance and cell seeding efficiency. Acta Biomater 7:1009–1018. doi:10.1016/j.actbio.2010.11.003

22. Pandithevan P, Saravana Kumar G (2009) Personalised bone tissue engineering scaffold with controlled architecture using fractal tool paths in layered manufacturing. Virt Phys Prototyp 4:165–180. doi:10.1080/17452750903055512

23. Kou XY, Tan ST (2010) A simple and effective geometric representation for irregular porous structure modeling. Comput Aided Des 42:930–941. doi:10.1016/j.cad.2010.06.006

24. Sun W, Starly B, Nam J, Darling A (2005) Bio-CAD modeling and its applications in computer-aided tissue engineering. Comput Aided Des 37:1097–1114. doi:10.1016/j.cad.2005.02.002

25. Pandithevan P, Kumar GS (2009) Reconstruction of subject-specific human femoral bone model with cortical porosity data using macro-CT. Virt Phys Prototyp 4:115–129

26. Chen Z, Su Z, Ma S, Wu X, Luo Z (2007) Biomimetic modeling and three-dimension reconstruction of the artificial bone. Comput Methods Programs Biomed 88:123–130

27. Tellis BC, Szivek JA, Bliss CL, Margolis DS, Vaidyanathan RK, Calvert P (2008) Trabecular scaffolds created using micro CT guided fused deposition modeling. Mater Sci Eng C 28:171–178

28. Leong KF, Chua CK, Sudarmadji N, Yeong Y (2008) Engineering functionally graded tissue engineering scaffolds. J Mech Behav Biomed Mater 1:140–152

29. Chen Y, Cadman J, Zhou S, Li Q (2011) Computer-aided design and fabrication of biomimetic materials and scaffold micro-structures. Adv Mater Res 213:628–632

30. Lacroix D, Planell JA, Prendergast PJ (2009) Computer-aided design and finite-element modelling of biomaterial scaffolds for bone tissue engineering. Philos Trans R Soc A 367:1993–2009

31. Sandino C, Planell JA, Lacroix D (2008) A finite element study of mechanical stimuli in scaffolds for bone tissue engineering. J Biomech 41:1005–1014

32. Olivares AL, Marsal E, Planell JA, Lacroix D (2009) Finite element study of scaffold architecture design and culture conditions for tissue engineering. Biomaterials 30:6142–6149
33. Cahill S, Lohfeld S, McHugh PE (2009) Finite element predictions compared to experimental results for the effective modulus of bone tissue engineering scaffolds fabricated by selective laser sintering. J Mater Sci, Mater Med 20:1255–1262
34. Rezwan K, Chen QZ, Blaker JJ, Boccaccini AR (2006) Biodegradable and bioactive porous polymer/inorganic composite scaffolds for bone tissue engineering. Biomaterials 27:3413–3431
35. Bendsøe MP, Sigmund O (2003) Topology optimization: theory, methods, and applications. Springer, London
36. Almeida HdE, Bártolo PJ (2010) Virtual topological optimisation of scaffolds for rapid prototyping. Med Eng Phys 32:775–782
37. Boccaccio A, Ballini A, Pappalettere C, Tullo D, Cantore S, Desiate A (2011) Finite element method (FEM), mechanobiology and biomimetic scaffolds in bone tissue engineering. Int J Biol Sci 7:112–132
38. Chen Y, Zhou S, Li Q (2011) Microstructure design of biodegradable scaffold and its effect on tissue regeneration. Biomaterials 32:5003–5014. doi:10.1016/j.biomaterials.2011.03.064
39. Byrne DP, Lacroix D, Planell JA, Kelly DJ, Prendergast PJ (2007) Simulation of tissue differentiation in a scaffold as a function of porosity, Young's modulus and dissolution rate: application of mechanobiological models in tissue engineering. Biomaterials 28:5544–5554. doi:10.1016/j.biomaterials.2007.09.003
40. Michell AGM (1904) The limits of economy of material in frame-structures. Philos Mag Ser 6 8:589–597. doi:10.1080/14786440409463229
41. Culmann K (1866) Die graphische Statik. Meyer & Zeller, Zürich
42. Jang IG, Kim IY (2008) Computational study of Wolff's law with trabecular architecture in the human proximal femur using topology optimization. J Biomech 41:2353–2361
43. Rainer A, Giannitelli SM, Accoto D, De Porcellinis S, Guglielmelli E, Trombetta M (2011) Load-adaptive scaffold architecturing: a bioinspired approach to the design of porous additively manufactured scaffolds with optimized mechanical properties. Ann Biomed Eng 40:966–975. doi:10.1007/s10439-011-0465-4
44. Papini M, Zdero R, Schemitsch EH, Zalzal P (2007) The biomechanics of human femurs in axial and torsional loading: comparison of finite element analysis, human cadaveric femurs, and synthetic femurs. J Biomech Eng 129:12–19
45. Keaveny TM, Guo XE, Wachtel EF, McMahon TA, Hayes WC (1994) Trabecular bone exhibits fully linear elastic behavior and yields at low strains. J Biomech 27:1127–1136
46. McIntosh L, Cordell JM, Wagoner Johnson AJ (2009) Impact of bone geometry on effective properties of bone scaffolds. Acta Biomater 5:680–692
47. Viceconti M, Bellingeri L, Cristofolini L, Toni A (1998) A comparative study on different methods of automatic mesh generation on human femurs. Med Eng Phys 20:1–10
48. Koch JC (1917) The laws of bone architecture. Am J Anat 21:177–298
49. Hobbie RK, Roth BJ (2007) Intermediate physics for medicine and biology. Springer, Berlin
50. Pálfi P (2002) Locally orthotropic femur model. J Comput Appl Mech 5:103–115
51. Pandithevan P, Kumar GS (2010) Finite element analysis of a personalized femoral scaffold with designed microarchitecture. Proc Inst Mech Eng H 224:877–889. doi:10.1243/09544119jeim633

Rational Design of Artificial Cellular Niches for Tissue Engineering

Ana Sancho, Javier Aldazabal, Alberto Rainer, and Elena M. De-Juan-Pardo

Abstract Tissue Engineering is a promising emerging field that studies the intrinsic regenerative potential of the human body and uses it to restore functionality of damaged organs or tissues unable of self-healing due to illness or ageing. In order to achieve regeneration using Tissue Engineering strategies, it is first necessary to study the properties of the native tissue and determine the cause of tissue failure; second, to identify an optimum population of cells capable of restoring its functionality; and third, to design and manufacture a cellular microenvironment in which those specific cells are directed towards the desired cellular functions. The design of the artificial cellular niche has a tremendous importance, because cells will feel and respond to both its biochemical and biophysical properties very differently. In particular, the artificial niche will act as a physical scaffold for the cells, allowing their three-dimensional spatial organization; also, it will provide mechanical stability to the artificial construct; and finally, it will supply biochemical and mechanical cues to control cellular growth, migration, differentiation and synthesis of natural extracellular matrix. During the last decades, many scientists have made great contributions to the field of Tissue Engineering. Even though this research has frequently been accompanied by vast investments during extended periods of time, yet too often these efforts have not been enough to translate the advances into new clinical therapies. More and more scientists in this field are aware of the need of rational experimental designs before carrying out complex, expensive and time-consuming in vitro and in vivo trials. This review highlights the importance of computer modeling and novel biofabrication techniques as critical key players for a rational design of artificial cellular niches in Tissue Engineering.

A. Sancho · J. Aldazabal · A. Rainer
Tissue Engineering and Biomaterials Unit, CEIT and Tecnun, University of Navarra, Manuel de Lardizábal 15, 20018 San Sebastián, Spain

E.M. De-Juan-Pardo (✉)
Institute of Health and Biomedical Innovation, Queensland University of Technology, 60 Musk Ave, 4059 Kelvin Grove, Queensland, Australia
e-mail: elena.juanpardo@qut.edu.au

P.R. Fernandes, P.J. Bártolo (eds.), *Tissue Engineering*,
Computational Methods in Applied Sciences 31, DOI 10.1007/978-94-007-7073-7_7,
© Springer Science+Business Media Dordrecht 2014

1 The Importance of the Cellular Niche in Tissue Engineering

Tissue Engineering is a promising emerging field that studies the intrinsic regenerative potential of the human body and uses it to restore functionality of damaged organs or tissues unable of self-healing due to illness or ageing.

Every living cell is affected by the surrounding microenvironment, known as the extracellular matrix (ECM) [1]. Many recent studies reveal that biophysical and biochemical features of the ECM such as stiffness, biochemical composition and matrix topography can influence and also dictate cellular response [2–4]. The cellular niche is also relevant for modulating cellular forces exerted on the ECM [5]; these forces activate specific signaling pathways, which further trigger transcription factors that control gene expression in the nucleus [6]. This effect, known as mechanotransduction, affects cell adhesion, proliferation, motility, differentiation and apoptosis [7, 8].

Therefore, the design of controlled artificial cellular niches has a tremendous importance to direct cells towards specific functions. Using Tissue Engineering strategies, the artificial niche will have to recapitulate the natural ECM. As a result, the engineered construct will serve as a physical scaffold for the cells, allowing their three-dimensional (3D) spatial organization; it will also ensure the mechanical stability of the whole construct; finally, it will provide biochemical and biophysical cues which will have an impact on cellular growth, migration, differentiation and synthesis of natural ECM.

For a rational design of artificial ECMs, we propose to start by studying the properties of the native tissue. Characterizing healthy tissues and identifying their differences compared to damaged ones has shown potential to facilitate disease detection and development of novel targets for regenerative medicine [9, 10]. Special attention should be paid to the biophysical aspects (biochemical composition and mechanical properties) as well as the macro-, micro- and nanoscopic structure of the ECM [11, 12], since both have remarkable effects on cellular responses.

During the last decades, great contributions have been made by a growing scientific community in the field of Tissue Engineering. Although this field has required—and still does—substantial economical investments during extended periods of time, these funds have not always been sufficient to translate research advances into new clinical therapies. To a greater extent, scientists in this field are aware of the need of more rationale before carrying out complex, expensive and time-consuming in vitro and in vivo trials.

This chapter will recall the importance of the development of better models, highlighting computer modeling and novel biofabrication techniques as critical key players for a rational design of artificial cellular niches in Tissue Engineering. It will also review the latest efforts towards the development of human-on-chip models thanks to the progression of microfluidics.

2 Characterization of Natural Microenvironments

2.1 Main Components of the Natural ECM

The natural cellular microenvironment contains both intrinsic and extrinsic signals that regulate cellular functions: quiescence, self-renewal, proliferation, differentiation, motility, and apoptosis. This microenvironment varies in its characteristics depending on the tissue it is part of [1]. Nevertheless, common features of cellular microenvironments can be recognized: they are 3D complexes consisting of: (a) a cellular compartment, where different types of cells are found (e.g. for the bone marrow: fibroblasts, osteoblasts, endothelial cells, stromal cells, etc.) [13]; (b) an ECM component, which acts as a dynamic support for cell anchorage and intercellular communication [14]; and (c) a soluble component, which includes cytokines, growth factors, metalloproteinases, etc. that contribute to matrix remodeling and cell fate regulation [15].

In the ECM, different types of proteins are found, such as collagen, fibronectin, laminin, vitronectin, and tenascin, together with a wide variety of proteoglycans like hyaluronan, aggrecan, and decorin. Around 28 different molecules of collagen, the most extensive protein in vertebrates, have already been found. Among them, type I–III, V, and XI are triple helices of fibril structures (Fig. 1).

There is a wide variety of types of ECM in vertebrates, depending on tissues. The main tissues in vertebrates are nerve, muscle, blood, lymphoid, epithelial and connective tissues. Among them, epithelial and connective tissues are the most distinct ones in terms of cell density and characteristics of the ECM. In the former, cells are abundant and form a cell sheet that endures most of the mechanical stresses in

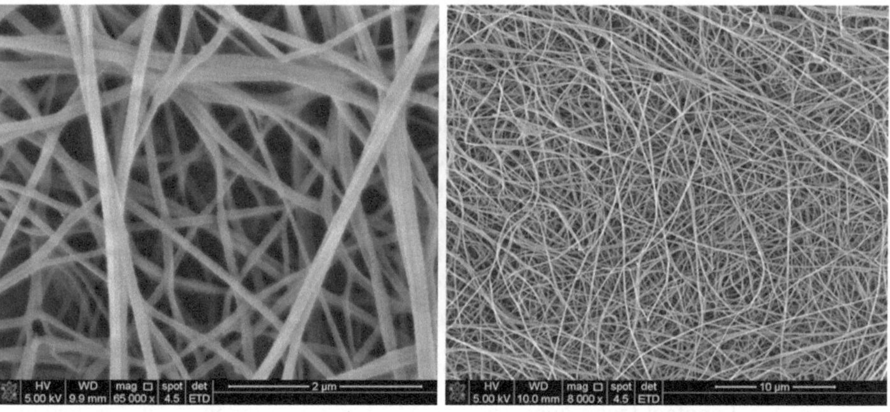

Fig. 1 Images of collagen hydrogels of 0.5 mg/mL (PureCol®, Advanced BioMatrix). *Left*: Triple helix in type I collagen fibrils using an equipment that combines a Focused Iom Beam (FIB) module with a Field Emission Gun (FE)-Scanning Electron Microscope (SEM) (FIB/FESEM, Quanta 3D™ DualBeam™ FEI). *Right*: Micrograph of fribillar type-I collagen taken with the same FIB/FESEM instrument. Images courtesy of Laboratory of Tissue Engineering, CEIT, San Sebastian, Spain

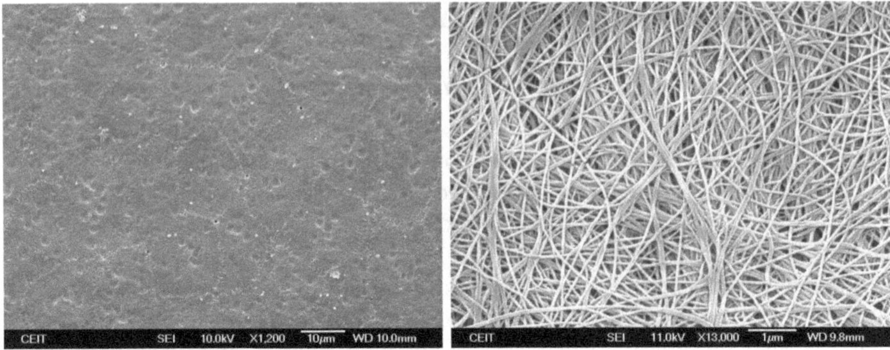

Fig. 2 Micrograph showing the epithelium of an amniotic membrane (*left*) and the stroma underlying the basal lamina of an amniotic membrane (*right*). Micrographs were acquired with a FESEM instrument, JEOL JSM-7100F. Samples courtesy of Laboratory of Cell Therapy, University Clinic of Navarra, Pamplona, Spain

the tissue (Fig. 2 left), while anchoring to the underlying basal lamina formed by the ECM, also known as basement membrane. By contrast, the connective tissue is characterized by a sparse cell distribution and abundant ECM, where cells exert forces (Fig. 2 right). Epithelial tissues form barriers for the control of fluid exchange and they usually rest on a connective tissue that facilitates its adhesion to more specialized tissues [16].

2.2 Characterization Techniques

We have highlighted the importance of a precise characterization of the natural niche for a rational design of artificial ECMs. In the following, a brief review of the main characterization techniques will be provided.

Traditionally, biochemical characterization tools have played a major role when studying the maturation or functionality of the tissues. Basic techniques used in this field, together with histology and immunohistochemistry, are immunoblotting and PCR analysis, which facilitate the quantification of proteins and gene expression, respectively. In this section, we will give special attention to other techniques suitable for a thorough characterization of the mechanical properties and architecture of the natural ECM. In particular, we will emphasize the advantages of microscopy as a powerful tool to study morphological features. In addition, we will recommend the use of local contact techniques, such as AFM and nanoindentation, for the characterization of the mechanical properties of natural ECMs.

Microscopy is an essential characterization tool widely used in many fields of research, either in its many variations of light microscopy (phase contrast, bright field, fluorescence, etc.), confocal microscopy, two-photon microscopy, Scanning Electron Microscopy (SEM) or Atomic Force Microscopy (AFM). The contributions of

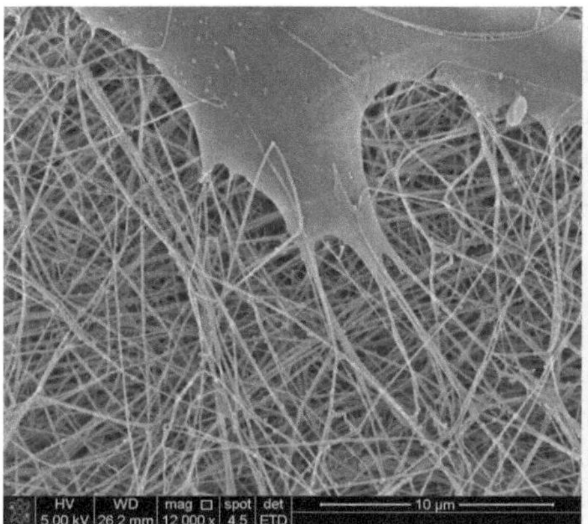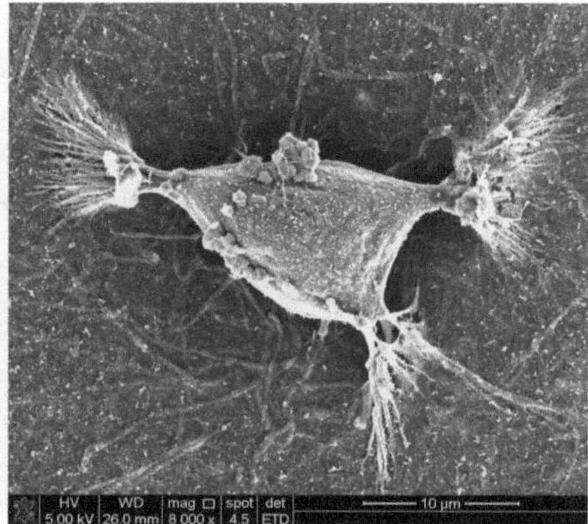

Fig. 3 *Left*: Detailed image of an Adipose-Derived Stem Cell (ADSC) cultured on a collagen hydrogel, where the alignment of fibrils is clearly visible around the cell-matrix adhesion sites. Micrograph obtained using a FIB-FESEM instrument (FEI Quanta 3D™ DualBeam™). *Right*: FIB-FESEM micrograph of an ADSC cultured on a collagen-agarose gel; alignment of collagen fibrils is also remarkable at the main adhesion sites. Images courtesy of Laboratory of Tissue Engineering and Biomaterials, CEIT, San Sebastian, Spain

the last two above-mentioned variations of microscopy have been particularly relevant for the nanostructural and mechanical characterization of the natural tissue in Tissue Engineering.

SEM allows for the acquisition of very high magnification images; and even more, Field Emission Gun (FE)-SEM instruments, which are widely used for the nanostructural characterization of surfaces [17]. Figure 3 shows two examples of cells cultured on fibrous scaffolds. Moreover, these electron microscopes can be combined with a Focused Ion Beam (FIB) module, which allows for high precision milling of samples. As a result, 3D nanostructural analysis can be performed. The main drawback of this technique is the need of working with dehydrated samples, which enhances the risk of altering the microstructure during sample preparation. To overcome this limitation, cryogenic modules have been developed which do not require dehydration of samples.

Atomic Force Microscopy (AFM) and other local contact methods, such as nanoindentation, are recently drawing attention for the mechanical characterization of biological tissues [18]. In these tests, both the load and displacement of a small probe, the indenter tip, are continuously monitored as the probe is loaded onto the surface of interest. Local contact methods are ideal for probing small samples, local gradients and heterogeneities in biological materials; they are also powerful tools for examining hierarchical and multiscale organization of cells and tissues. In addition, no extensive sample preparation is required prior to mechanical testing, in contrast to other techniques. Finally, most nanoindentation instruments allow purposeful exploration of a variety of different deformation modes by changing experimental time scale, indenter tip geometry and loading conditions. Although earliest applications of these techniques had been designed for the analysis of metallic and ceramic materials, during the last decade novel bio-AFM equipments have been developed (e.g. Asylum Research MFP-3D-BIO Atomic Force Microscope System; Nanonics Hydra BioAFM; JPK Instruments NanoWizard 3 BioAFM; Bruker BioScope Catalyst AFM) to work with living cells at physiological conditions and even under flow conditions, while the mechanical testing is performed. Consequently, their application is not restricted to hard materials anymore, opening a new field for the analysis of mechanical properties of cells themselves [19, 20].

3 In Vitro Biomimetic Models: From Tissues to Models

The manufacture of physiologically relevant in vitro biomimetic models is critical for both the development and validation of novel products in Tissue Engineering.

3.1 Controlling Cell-Cell and Cell-Matrix Interactions

In the previous section, we have highlighted the importance of a thorough characterization of the natural tissue that wants to be replaced. In this section, we want to emphasize the importance of studying the key cell-cell and cell-matrix interactions that will take part during the regeneration process: i.e., how a particular cell type will respond to the design parameters of a certain scaffold, such as rigidity, microstructural arrangement, surface chemistry, etc., and how it will interact with other neighbor cells present.

3.1.1 Cellular Response to Mechanical and Topographical Cues

As we have already described, organs are formed by tissues, which are mainly composed of cells and the ECM. Certain mechanical properties are associated to every healthy tissue, and every tissue cell is adapted to it, ensuring homeostasis [21, 22]. For instance, tissues such as brain or adipose tissue are more compliant than bone or cartilage. In the case of epithelial cancers, tumors are stiffer than the surrounding tissue and might be detected through physical palpation, as a rigid mass residing within a compliant tissue. Monitoring of tumors based on rigidity maps is widespread, but the relationship between tissue rigidity and tumor behavior at the molecular level is still unclear [23]. It has been observed that tumor rigidity could influence treatment efficacy, enhancing tumor metastasis. In addition, cells adhere more strongly and migrate faster on stiffer substrates [24]. Tumor progression leads to variations in the ECM organization and stiffness of the tumor mass itself; moreover, it also induces changes in the viscoelastic properties of the stromal cells associated with the tumor [25, 26].

Many studies have been performed in order to define the effect that matrix stiffness has in the differentiation of stem cells towards specific phenotypes [27, 28].

It has already been stated that, for mesenchymal stem cell cultures, soft matrices that mimic mechanical properties of the brain, are able to induce neurogenesis—i.e. active production of new neurons and other brain cells—while rigid matrices that mimic bone rigidity induce osteogenesis, i.e. formation of bone tissue [27]. Apart from the matrix stiffness, the elastic properties of the cells also undergo variations during the differentiation process and maturation [29, 30].

Concerning the surface topography of the microenvironment around the cells, it has been established that the nano-topography of the substrate has a remarkable influence on cell behavior. In the case of stem cells, nano-topography can contribute in undifferentiated cell proliferation or in directing differentiation into a specific cell lineage [2, 31].

3.1.2 Biofabrication Techniques

Novel biofabrication techniques offer exceptional promises for the development of biomimetic in vitro devices, which combine controlled microenvironments with multiple scaffolds and cellular configurations [32–36].

Among all biofabrication techniques, soft lithography has shown a great potential for the manufacture of miniaturized in vitro systems with unique spatio-temporal resolution. This technique can process a wide variety of polymeric materials [37, 38], from which Polydimethylsiloxane (PDMS) has been the most extensively used for the manufacture of controlled microfluidic devices [39]. PDMS is transparent, reasonably cheap, straightforward to mold and easy to bond to different materials, such as glass, polystyrene (PS) or PDMS itself. Remarkably, PS is also currently arising as one of the most appropriate materials for the manufacture of in vitro microdevices due to its excellent compatibility for cellular experiments [40].

Soft lithography is a non-photolitographic method that transfers the geometry of a photolithographically-obtained mold (*master*), endowed with micro or nanoscale patterns and fabricated with e.g. SU-8 epoxy-based photoresist, into the desired polymeric material, typically PDMS. A standard soft-lithographic process includes two main fabrication steps: first, manufacture of the SU-8 master; and second, geometry transfer to the PDMS. For the manufacture of the master, a photoresist is spun onto a silicon or glass wafer until forming a continuous thin layer and then is exposed to ultraviolet (UV) light through a mask of well-defined geometry containing the designed features; afterwards, the development of the photoresist gives rise to the SU-8 master. The master geometry is easily transferred on PDMS by pouring liquid PDMS on the master and heat-curing it to obtain a solid rubber. The obtained PDMS *replica* can be peeled off from the master and bonded to a glass slide sealing the channels and forming the final microdevice. Geometrical features of the microdevices can be adjusted to create patterned cell cultures, microfluidic channels at cellular or subcellular scales, generate chemical gradients of chemoattractant substances, etc., making soft lithography a very versatile technology for the manufacture of miniaturized controlled biomimetic in vitro models.

Together with soft lithography, novel bioprinting technologies are also outstanding biofabrication techniques developed to recapitulate the intrinsic complexity of native tissues in vitro [41–44]. Very briefly, bioprinting technologies, based on the principles of rapid prototyping, manufacture complex constructs made of polymeric materials, cells or both with a particular spatial organization that mimic a certain tissue [41].

3.2 Artificial Microenvironments: Synthesis and Manufacture

In order to produce realistic in vitro models, it is advisable to be familiarized with the most recent synthesis and manufacturing processes of artificial microenvironments. Thus, special attention will be drawn to the last advances in the synthesis of biopolymers for the fabrication of ECM surrogates, alone or in combination with inorganic particles or bioactive molecules.

A plethora of biocompatible materials—both natural and synthetic—have been investigated for the fabrication of artificial microenvironments. Natural polymers, comprising collagen and its derivatives, fibrin, and a wide selection of polysaccharides (hyaluronan, alginate, chitosan, agarose) have been used for their biochemical similarity with natural components of ECM and for their capacity to form hydrogels to encapsulate cells [45–47].

Among synthetic materials, aliphatic polyesters, such as poly(L-lactide), poly(glycolide), poly(ε-caprolactone), and their co-polymers represent the most popular biomaterials [48]. Polyurethanes represent another widely investigated class of materials, whose mechanical and chemical properties can be tuned by proper selection of the starting oligomers [49].

Synthetic polymers can be modified in order to mimic specific properties of natural ECM, such as specific cell adhesion, degradation by proteolytic processes involved in cell migration and tissue remodeling, and the ability to control cell functions. The possibility to independently modulate physical and biomolecular signaling of biomaterials open new scenarios in the re-creation—into controlled in vitro settings—of artificial analogs of the ECM to simulate the tissue niche.

PEG-based hydrogels represent the gold standard for such an application due to their intrinsic hydrophilicity and resistance to protein absorption. Such materials provide a bioinert backbone on which the desired biofunctionality can be built. Mann and coworkers [50] have synthesized a photopolymerizable PEG-based gel with the insertion of adhesion peptides sequences (e.g. RGD), as well as metalloproteinase-cleavable peptide domains, in order to create a synthetic ECM analog. Similar results were obtained by Miller et al., who obtained PEG-based gels with tunable MMP-sensitivity by introducing peptide domains with several degrees of modifications with respect to native collagen [51].

Acrylate-endcapped PEG represents a convenient starting material to obtain photopolymerizable gels. Polymerization can be performed not only by UV irradiation, but also under visible light, using mild photocatalysts, that are compatible with cell life (e.g. eosin Y). Therefore, microencapsulation of living cells within the gel phase can be performed [52].

StarPEG-heparin hydrogels were tailored for storage and controlled release of high affinity GAG-binding proteins, in a fashion that closely resembles the mechanisms occurring within natural tissue [53].

3.3 Natural Microenvironments: Decellularized ECMs

Decellularization of natural ECMs is particularly relevant within the field of organ engineering, where whole-organ development is pursued. Despite the remarkable achievements and extensive work already performed by tissue engineers in heart, kidney, pancreas and lung regeneration, a complete functionality of the whole organs has not yet been reached [54]. The first step in this process consists on the removal of every cell in a donor organ by the perfusion of detergents, proteases and chemicals; the aggressiveness of the process can damage the structure and composition of the resulting acellular 3D matrix, thus, altering the host response of these scaffolds regarding to the organ reconstruction [55]. In the second step of the process, a selection of cell populations are seeded in the acellular matrix, considering the different cell types that are present in complex tissues and organs, in order to regenerate every structure such as the parenchyma and vasculature. Many alternatives are being evaluated as potential cell sources, including pluripotent stem cells, adult progenitor cells or, in particular cases, tissue-derived differentiated cells; moreover, autologous versus allogeneic cell sources are under study [56]. Finally, in order to enhance the repopulation of the construct, specific culture conditions, adequate for the organ in reconstruction, must be ensured. This is commonly achieved by means of bioreactors, which can perfuse the culture media in the construct for the nutrient and oxygen supply, and they can even provide the system with biophysical stimulation as mechanical or electrical stimuli.

3.4 Model Implementation: Tissues- and Organs-on-a-Chip

In this section, a selection of a few significant examples of model implementations of *tissues-* and *organs-on-a-chip* will be brought up from the literature to illustrate the great potential of in vitro microdevices for Tissue Engineering.

Moraes and co-workers have recently used the term *tissue-on-a-chip* to identify any micro-engineered system with controlled properties that achieves the formation of tissue constructs using cells, soluble factors, fluid shear or perfused culture medium [57]. Similarly, *organ-on-a-chip* is used to designate a more complex microengineered system that is able to recapitulate the in vivo milieu at an organ level, frequently applying microscale compartmentalization strategies [57]. Their work nicely reviews the last advances towards developing functional *organs-on-a-chip*.

Work conducted at the Griffith Laboratory reported as early as in 2002 on the design, fabrication, and performance of a bioreactor for both morphogenesis of 3D tissue structures under continuous perfusion and tissue growth observation by in situ light microscopy [58]; their system was successfully applied to study the functional viability of primary rat hepatocytes maintained in this microarray bioreactor [59]. Research directed by Vacanti pioneered the concept of engineering a vasculature using microfabrication techniques, when they reported the formation of endothelium-on-a-chip using a vascular geometry in microfabricated PDMS [60]. Many other authors have also worked using similar concepts. For example, Huh and co-workers developed a human airway epithelia-on-a-chip and showed cellular level lung injury under pathologic liquid plug flows [61]. More recently, Lam et al. have developed a novel method to obtain muscle, by first templating myoblast alignment on rigid microtopographically patterned surfaces and then transferring myotubes into a degradable hydrogel that allowed for self-organization of the cells into a functional, 3D and free-standing construct [62]. Recent research performed at the Ingber Laboratory remarkably accomplished the reconstruction of lung-on-a-chip, where the critical functional alveolar capillary interface of the human lung was mimicked [63].

In summary, last advances towards the development of *organs-on-a-chip* have become a reality and mean a great hope for achieving an effective reduction in the number of animal studies and for faster and effective progression in Tissue Engineering.

4 In Silico Models: Design and Validation

As stated before, timeframes required to translate Tissue Engineering products form bench to bedside are very long and require extensive in vitro and in vivo validation steps, thus increasing the overall costs of the final product. It has been estimated that the average time for the development of a Tissue Engineering product can go up to 10 years [64]. Therefore, substantial investments are required, in terms of laboratory equipment, men power and validation tests, until the commercialization of the product is reached.

In this framework, it is clear how in silico experiments, based on accurate computer models, could help reduce the overall costs of final Tissue Engineering products in a drastic way. In this section, novel in silico modeling techniques applicable to simulate the manufacturing process of a scaffold and its degradation process in the body will be briefly reviewed.

4.1 Simulation of Manufacturing Processes of Scaffolds

Manufacturing process is crucial in determining scaffolds characteristics. Among the broad variety of techniques developed to manufacture customized scaffolds, additive manufacturing and electrospinning will be highlighted in this section. Additive manufacturing techniques, specially extrusion-based ones, are widely used to produce tailor-maid structures with relatively thick polymeric fibers. The diameter of these fibers ranges from several dozens to hundreds of microns. These techniques are based on a computer controlled micro-extruder that dispenses a fluid polymer following a predefined path that solidify once it has been deposited [65]. Another standard method used for manufacturing fibrous scaffolds is electrospinning. This technique is used to produce randomly placed nanometric fibers. The process starts when a polymeric solution is placed into a syringe, and a high voltage is applied between the syringe needle and a collector plate. As the solution exits from the needle, the electric field accelerates the jet and shrinks its diameter down to nanometers [66].

4.1.1 Additive Manufacturing

The manufacture of scaffolds using additive manufacturing starts with the design of the microstructure in a CAD environment. Modeling complex microstructures created by this method is not always an easy task. A straightforward way to model scaffolds produced with additive-manufacturing-based approaches consists of using the same computational information that has been created to print the scaffold as an input to generate a virtual scaffold [67].

In some cases, it may be interesting to model the manufacturing process itself, directly generating in silico digital volumes with a certain disposition of the fibers so that the virtual scaffold matches the microstructure produced experimentally by other researchers [68]. Also, it might be practical to use data from computer tomography imaging of real scaffolds as input for the generation of scaffolds in silico [69]. The generation of those digitalized 3D microstructures could be used to measure or predict some physical and mechanical properties of the scaffold related to its microstructure, or even for degradation studies.

4.1.2 Electrospinning

Modeling the generation of scaffolds by electrospinning is definitely more challenging than by rapid prototyping. Scaffolds produced by electrospinning are fibrous polymer-based materials where the arrangement of fibers and their diameters are difficult to predict. Many parameters, such as polymer/solvent ratio, molecular weight of the polymer, viscosity, surface tension, conductivity, applied voltage, flow rate, needle-collector distance, among others, have an impact on the final geometry of the scaffold [70]. In the following lines, a method to model electrospun microstructures in a very realistic fashion will be presented. As an example obtained applying this method, Fig. 4 left shows a real electrospun microstructure and Fig. 4 right shows a modeled scaffold generated for degradation studies.

If studies are going to be performed in very small regions of the scaffold, it is possible to presume that fibers have a constant diameter, are locally straight and randomly oriented in different layers. Using these assumptions, some authors have

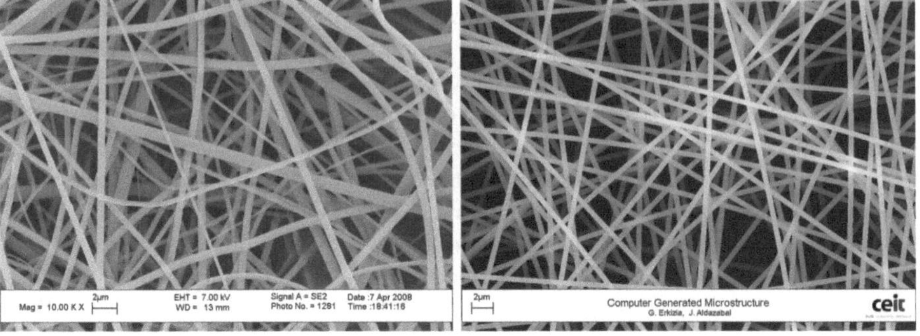

Fig. 4 *Left*: SEM micrograph of a poly(L-lactide) (PLLA) electrospun scaffold. Image courtesy of Laboratory of Tissue Engineering and Biomaterials, CEIT, San Sebastian, Spain. *Right*: Computer-generated microstructure of an electrospun scaffold modeled to study the relationship between the geometry of the scaffold and its degradation rate [71]

already developed a computational model to predict the mechanical properties of non-woven scaffolds [72], the degradation of PLLA scaffolds [71] or the filtration of nanoparticles in electrospun mats [73].

Other authors have focused their attention on the modeling of the electrospinning process itself, developing numerical models capable of predicting the path that an electrospun fiber will follow from the needle to the collector [74, 75]. Their input parameters are the real physical parameters that govern the electrospinning manufacturing process. These models consider electrospun fibers as poly-lines and calculate all the stresses, stretches and velocities in the nodes, being able to reproduce very realistically the final fiber paths. These models are, however, computationally very demanding, so that they are not useful when generation of large microstructures is required [76].

4.2 Modeling Microstructural Properties

Once a realistic microstructure of a scaffold has been generated in silico, it is possible to develop computational models to study or deduce some important properties of the scaffold, such as stiffness, permeability or degradation rate of the fibers. Only when these models have been validated against empirical measurements, they are suitable for the rational design of scaffolds in a more efficient way.

4.2.1 Mechanical and Structural Properties

The requirements of a scaffold in terms of mechanical properties have to be completely elucidated in view of a tissue engineering application. As previously explained, a scaffold has to provide sufficient mechanical stability during service and

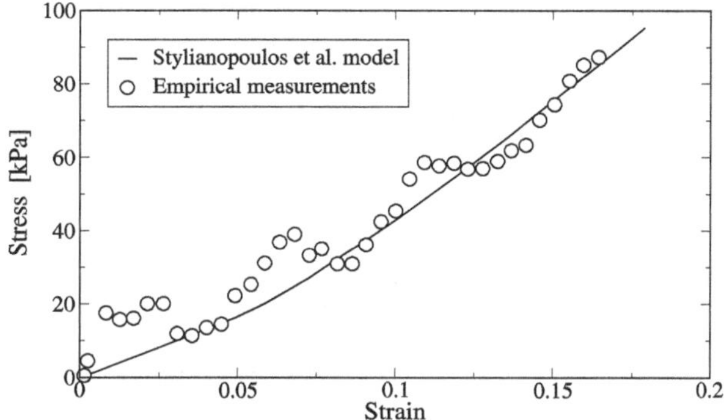

Fig. 5 Elasto-plastic response of an electrospun scaffold measured empirically by tensile test (*circles*) and in silico predicted using a poly-line/spring model (*solid line*) [72]

show a certain mechanical response to stimulate the proliferation of cells until the newly regenerated tissue is formed.

The use of finite element method for predicting the mechanical properties of rapid-prototyping-produced scaffolds is straightforward, as these microstructures are usually simple, with well-defined geometries [77]. Simulating microstructures produced by electrospinning, however, becomes much more complex, as fibers are randomly located. Due to scaffolds random morphologies, it would be very inaccurate to work with a small representative volume element (RVE); conversely, large RVEs must be used. This implies that such entities cannot be handled in an efficient way using finite element codes by average-performance computers. New smarter models have been recently proposed to solve this problem, where electrospun microstructures are handled as poly-lines [72, 78]. These models replace the poly-line by a sequence of springs, assuming that the spring constant describes the elastic modulus of the polymer; they also use a "bond angle potential" to reproduce its flexural stiffness. Results obtained using this model for non-woven porous scaffold have been able to perfectly match empirical measurements, as shown in Fig. 5.

4.2.2 Perfusion/Vascularization

Cell proliferation inside a porous scaffold needs for an adequate supply of oxygen and nutrients; and vascularization of a scaffold involves cell migration. Therefore, any realistic computational model used in Tissue Engineering should implement diffusion of oxygen, nutrients, wastes, etc. throughout the physiological medium that wets the entire scaffold. This requirement makes necessary to study and understand diffusion through a scaffold.

Very important properties, such as porosity, pressure drop or permeability, will change depending on scaffold microstructure. Several authors have developed different 3D models to infer the dependence of such properties from geometric cues. Usually all these studies have been conducted using standard computational fluid dynamics (CFD) environments, such as Fluent [73, 79, 80]. Recently, other authors have also used similar models to design and optimize microfluidic assays combining 2D and 3D cell cultures [81]. Lately, some other authors have developed even

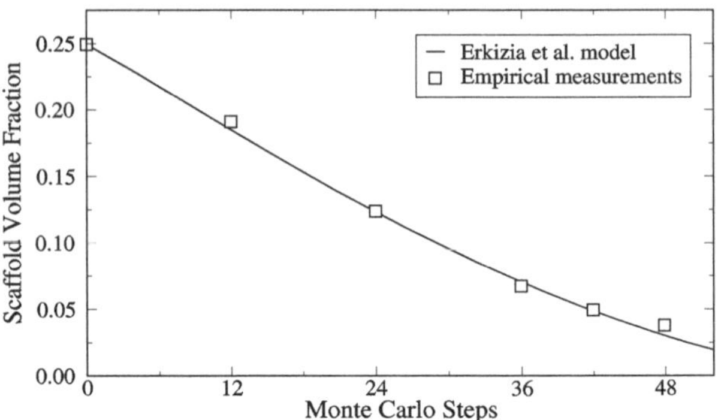

Fig. 6 Degradation of a PCL/TCP scaffold empirically measured by Lam et al. (*boxes*) and predicted by Erkizia et al. (*solid line*)

more complex mathematical models, using a set of coupled non-linear ordinary differential equations, which describe the evolution of the different tissue constituents inside scaffolds [82].

4.2.3 Scaffold Degradation/Drug Release

One of the main aims of Tissue Engineering consists in replacing the artificial scaffold with natural tissue. This replacement requires degradation of the scaffold to be timely compatible with the rate of tissue neo-formation.

For this reason, several authors have empirically measured and computer-modeled scaffold degradation rate. Using different 3D techniques, they have developed degradation models of additively-manufactured [83] and electrospun scaffolds [84], and even degradation of spherical particles [85, 86]. Figure 6 shows the degradation profile of an additively-manufactured scaffold as documented in Erkizia et al. [83].

In some cases it is interesting to introduce substances in the scaffold that will interact with the surrounding natural tissue, such as drugs, growth factors or vaccines. In these cases, the above-mentioned molecules are not released instantaneously but in a controlled manner, as the scaffold degrades.

This has also been the object of investigations by several authors who have faced these issues from many different perspectives. Some of the first one-dimensional models developed in the late '70s and early '80s were simple mathematical models that considered the diffusion from the surface of cylinders or spheres that contained a homogeneous distribution of drug inside [87, 88]. Nowadays, 3D models developed for degradation studies are capable to reproduce release profiles in real scaffolds. Using these models, it is possible to infer the influence of geometrical features such as fibers geometry or drug localization on the overall drug-release profile [89].

5 Concluding Remarks

We have emphasized the importance of a rational design of in vitro models to accelerate advances in Tissue Engineering. Such advances might benefit the coordinated efforts spent in different disciplines including (i) in silico modeling; (ii) fabrication of smart 3D systems (taking advantage of innovative biomimetic materials and/or biofabrication techniques); and (iii) development of miniaturized (microfluidic) controlled environments for in vitro experiments.

It is an opinion of the Authors that the most significant contributions in the field of Tissue Engineering are to be expected from multidisciplinary approaches merging competences across these domains.

References

1. Frantz C, Stewart KM, Weaver VM (2010) The extracellular matrix at a glance. J Cell Sci 123:4195–4200. doi:10.1242/jcs.023820
2. Oh J, Recknor JB, Recknor JC, Mallapragada SK, Sakaguchi DS (2009) Soluble factors from neocortical astrocytes enhance neuronal differentiation of neural progenitor cells from adult rat hippocampus on micropatterned polymer substrates. J Biomed Mater Res, Part A 91:575–585. doi:10.1002/jbm.a.32242
3. Nelson CM, Vanduijn MM, Inman JL, Fletcher DA, Bissell MJ (2006) Tissue geometry determines sites of mammary branching morphogenesis in organotypic cultures. Science 314:298–300. doi:10.1126/science.1131000
4. Mori H, Gjorevski N, Inman JL, Bissell MJ, Nelson CM (2009) Self-organization of engineered epithelial tubules by differential cellular motility. Proc Natl Acad Sci USA 106:14890–14895. doi:10.1073/pnas.0901269106
5. Discher DE, Janmey P, Wang YL (2005) Tissue cells feel and respond to the stiffness of their substrate. Science 310:1139–1143. doi:10.1126/science.1116995
6. Sarkar P, Rao BM (2009) Molecular aspects of cardiac differentiation in embryonic stem cells. Crit Rev Biomed Eng 37:283–320. doi:00f1eff12a65576b
7. Leong WS, Tay CY, Yu H, Li A, Wu SC, Duc DH, Lim CT, Tan LP (2010) Thickness sensing of hMSCs on collagen gel directs stem cell fate. Biochem Biophys Res Commun 401:287–292. doi:10.1016/j.bbrc.2010.09.052
8. Reilly GC, Engler AJ (2010) Intrinsic extracellular matrix properties regulate stem cell differentiation. J Biomech 43:55–62. doi:10.1016/j.jbiomech.2009.09.009
9. Gang Z, Qi Q, Jing C, Wang C (2009) Measuring microenvironment mechanical stress of rat liver during diethylnitrosamine induced hepatocarcinogenesis by atomic force microscope. Microsc Res Tech 72:672–678. doi:10.1002/jemt.20716
10. Dulinska I, Targosz M, Strojny W, Lekka M, Czuba P, Balwierz W, Szymonski M (2006) Stiffness of normal and pathological erythrocytes studied by means of atomic force microscopy. J Biochem Biophys Methods 66:1–11. doi:10.1016/j.jbbm.2005.11.003
11. Klein TJ, Malda J, Sah RL, Hutmacher DW (2009) Tissue engineering of articular cartilage with biomimetic zones. Tissue Eng, Part B Rev 15:143–157. doi:10.1089/ten.TEB.2008.0563
12. Vinatier C, Guicheux J, Daculsi G, Layrolle P, Weiss P (2006) Cartilage and bone tissue engineering using hydrogels. Biomed Mater Eng 16:S107–S113
13. Balakumaran A, Robey PG, Fedarko N, Landgren O (2010) Bone marrow microenvironment in myelomagenesis: its potential role in early diagnosis. Expert Rev Mol Diagn 10:465–480. doi:10.1586/erm.10.31

14. Schmeichel KL, Weaver VM, Bissell MJ (1998) Structural cues from the tissue microenvironment are essential determinants of the human mammary epithelial cell phenotype. J Mammary Gland Biol Neoplasia 3:201–213

15. Leibovici J, Itzhaki O, Huszar M, Sinai J (2011) The tumor microenvironment: Part 1. Immunotherapy 3:1367–1384. doi:10.2217/imt.11.111

16. Alberts B, Johnson A, Lewis J, Raff M, Roberts K, Walter P (2007) Molecular biology of the cell, 5th edn. Garland Science, New York

17. Raspanti M, Protasoni M, Manelli A, Guizzardi S, Mantovani V, Sala A (2006) The extracellular matrix of the human aortic wall: ultrastructural observations by FEG-SEM and by tapping-mode AFM. Micron 37:81–86. doi:10.1016/j.micron.2005.06.002

18. Oyen ML, Cook RF (2009) A practical guide for analysis of nanoindentation data. J Mech Behav Biomed Mater 2:396–407. doi:10.1016/j.jmbbm.2008.10.002

19. Lekka M, Gil D, Pogoda K, Dulinska-Litewka J, Jach R, Gostek J, Klymenko O, Prauzner-Bechcicki S, Stachura Z, Wiltowska-Zuber J, Okon K, Laidler P (2012) Cancer cell detection in tissue sections using AFM. Arch Biochem Biophys 518:151–156. doi:10.1016/j.abb.2011.12.013

20. Watanabe T, Kuramochi H, Takahashi A, Imai K, Katsuta N, Nakayama T, Fujiki H, Suganuma M (2012) Higher cell stiffness indicating lower metastatic potential in B16 melanoma cell variants and in (-)-epigallocatechin gallate-treated cells. J Cancer Res Clin Oncol. doi:10.1007/s00432-012-1159-5

21. Filas BA, Bayly PV, Taber LA (2011) Mechanical stress as a regulator of cytoskeletal contractility and nuclear shape in embryonic epithelia. Ann Biomed Eng 39:443–454. doi:10.1007/s10439-010-0171-7

22. Butcher A, Milner R, Ellis K, Watson JT, Horner A (2009) Interaction of platelet-rich concentrate with bone graft materials: an in vitro study. J Orthop Trauma 23:195–200; discussion 201–192. doi:10.1097/BOT.0b013e31819b35db

23. Suresh S (2007) Biomechanics and biophysics of cancer cells. Acta Biomater 3:413–438. doi:10.1016/j.actbio.2007.04.002

24. Guo WH, Frey MT, Burnham NA, Wang YL (2006) Substrate rigidity regulates the formation and maintenance of tissues. Biophys J 90:2213–2220. doi:10.1529/biophysj.105.070144

25. Baker EL, Lu J, Yu D, Bonnecaze RT, Zaman MH (2010) Cancer cell stiffness: integrated roles of three-dimensional matrix stiffness and transforming potential. Biophys J 99:2048–2057. doi:10.1016/j.bpj.2010.07.051

26. Ulrich TA, de Juan-Pardo EM, Kumar S (2009) The mechanical rigidity of the extracellular matrix regulates the structure, motility, and proliferation of glioma cells. Cancer Res 69:4167–4174. doi:10.1158/0008-5472.can-08-4859

27. Engler AJ, Sen S, Sweeney HL, Discher DE (2006) Matrix elasticity directs stem cell lineage specification. Cell 126:677–689. doi:10.1016/j.cell.2006.06.044

28. Engler AJ, Carag-Krieger C, Johnson CP, Raab M, Tang H-Y, Speicher DW, Sanger JW, Sanger JM, Discher DE (2008) Embryonic cardiomyocytes beat best on a matrix with heart-like elasticity: scar-like rigidity inhibits beating. J Cell Sci 121:3794–3802. doi:10.1242/jcs.029678

29. Titushkin I, Cho M (2007) Modulation of cellular mechanics during osteogenic differentiation of human mesenchymal stem cells. Biophys J 93:3693–3702. doi:10.1529/biophysj.107.107797

30. Collinsworth AM, Zhang S, Kraus WE, Truskey GA (2002) Apparent elastic modulus and hysteresis of skeletal muscle cells throughout differentiation. Am J Physiol, Cell Physiol 283:C1219–1227. doi:10.1152/ajpcell.00502.2001

31. Bratt-Leal AM, Carpenedo RL, McDevitt TC (2009) Engineering the embryoid body microenvironment to direct embryonic stem cell differentiation. Biotechnol Prog 25:43–51. doi:10.1002/btpr.139

32. Reese BE, Zheng S, Evans B, Datar RH, Thundat T, Lin HK (2010) Microfluidic device for studying tumor cell extravasation in cancer metastasis. In: Biomedical sciences and engineering conference (BSEC), 25–26 May 2010, pp 1–4. doi:10.1109/bsec.2010.5510818

33. Webster A, Dyer CE, Haswell SJ, Greenman J (2010) A microfluidic device for tissue biopsy culture and interrogation. Anal Methods 2:1005–1007. doi:10.1039/C0AY00293C
34. Nie FQ, Yamada M, Kobayashi J, Yamato M, Kikuchi A, Okano T (2007) On-chip cell migration assay using microfluidic channels. Biomaterials 28:4017–4022. doi:10.1016/j.biomaterials.2007.05.037
35. Saadi W, Wang SJ, Lin F, Jeon NL (2006) A parallel-gradient microfluidic chamber for quantitative analysis of breast cancer cell chemotaxis. Biomed Microdevices 8:109–118. doi:10.1007/s10544-006-7706-6
36. Cheng SY, Heilman S, Wasserman M, Archer S, Shuler ML, Wu M (2007) A hydrogel-based microfluidic device for the studies of directed cell migration. Lab Chip 7:763–769. doi:10.1039/b618463d
37. Chien R-D (2006) Hot embossing of microfluidic platform. Int Commun Heat Mass Transf 33:645–653. doi:10.1016/j.icheatmasstransfer.2006.01.017
38. Pu Q, Elazazy MS, Alvarez JC (2008) Label-free detection of heparin, streptavidin, and other probes by pulsed streaming potentials in plastic microfluidic channels. Anal Chem 80:6532–6536. doi:10.1021/ac8003117
39. Becker H, Gartner C (2008) Polymer microfabrication technologies for microfluidic systems. Anal Bioanal Chem 390:89–111. doi:10.1007/s00216-007-1692-2
40. Berthier E, Young EW, Beebe D (2012) Engineers are from PDMS-land, Biologists are from Polystyrenia. Lab Chip 12:1224–1237. doi:10.1039/c2lc20982a
41. Jakab K, Norotte C, Marga F, Murphy K, Vunjak-Novakovic G, Forgacs G (2010) Tissue engineering by self-assembly and bio-printing of living cells. Biofabrication 2:022001. doi:10.1088/1758-5082/2/2/022001
42. Schuurman W, Khristov V, Pot MW, van Weeren PR, Dhert WJ, Malda J (2011) Bioprinting of hybrid tissue constructs with tailorable mechanical properties. Biofabrication 3:021001. doi:10.1088/1758-5082/3/2/021001
43. Arai K, Iwanaga S, Toda H, Capi G, Nishiyama Y, Nakamura M (2011) Three-dimensional inkjet biofabrication based on designed images. Biofabrication 3:034113
44. Snyder JE, Hamid Q, Wang C, Chang R, Emami K, Wu H, Sun W (2011) Bioprinting cell-laden matrigel for radioprotection study of liver by pro-drug conversion in a dual-tissue microfluidic chip. Biofabrication 3:034112. doi:10.1088/1758-5082/3/3/034112
45. Donati I, Stredanska S, Silvestrini G, Vetere A, Marcon P, Marsich E, Mozetic P, Gamini A, Paoletti S, Vittur F (2005) The aggregation of pig articular chondrocyte and synthesis of extracellular matrix by a lactose-modified chitosan. Biomaterials 26:987–998. doi:10.1016/j.biomaterials.2004.04.015
46. Nair S, Remya NS, Remya S, Nair PD (2011) A biodegradable in situ injectable hydrogel based on chitosan and oxidized hyaluronic acid for tissue engineering applications. Carbohydr Polym 85:838–844. doi:10.1016/j.carbpol.2011.04.004
47. Kreger ST, Voytik-Harbin SL (2009) Hyaluronan concentration within a 3D collagen matrix modulates matrix viscoelasticity, but not fibroblast response. Matrix Biology 28:336–346. doi:10.1016/j.matbio.2009.05.001
48. Rainer A, Spadaccio C, Sedati P, De Marco F, Carotti S, Lusini M, Vadala G, Di Martino A, Morini S, Chello M, Covino E, Denaro V, Trombetta M (2011) Electrospun hydroxyapatite-functionalized PLLA scaffold: potential applications in sternal bone healing. Ann Biomed Eng 39:1882–1890. doi:10.1007/s10439-011-0289-2
49. Park D, Wu W, Wang Y (2011) A functionalizable reverse thermal gel based on a polyurethane/PEG block copolymer. Biomaterials 32:777–786. doi:10.1016/j.biomaterials.2010.09.044
50. Mann BK, Gobin AS, Tsai AT, Schmedlen RH, West JL (2001) Smooth muscle cell growth in photopolymerized hydrogels with cell adhesive and proteolytically degradable domains: synthetic ECM analogs for tissue engineering. Biomaterials 22:3045–3051.
51. Miller JS, Shen CJ, Legant WR, Baranski JD, Blakely BL, Chen CS (2010) Bioactive hydrogels made from step-growth derived PEG-peptide macromers. Biomaterials 31:3736–3743. doi:10.1016/j.biomaterials.2010.01.058

52. Bahney CS, Lujan TJ, Hsu CW, Bottlang M, West JL, Johnstone B (2011) Visible light photoinitiation of mesenchymal stem cell-laden bioresponsive hydrogels. Eur Cells Mater 22:43–55

53. Baumann L, Prokoph S, Gabriel C, Freudenberg U, Werner C, Beck-Sickinger AG (2012) A novel, biased-like SDF-1 derivative acts synergistically with starPEG-based heparin hydrogels and improves eEPC migration in vitro. J Control Release 162:68–75. doi:10.1016/j.jconrel.2012.04.049

54. Song JJ, Ott HC (2011) Organ engineering based on decellularized matrix scaffolds. Trends Mol Med 17:424–432. doi:10.1016/j.molmed.2011.03.005

55. Hoshiba T, Lu H, Kawazoe N, Chen G (2010) Decellularized matrices for tissue engineering. Expert Opin Biol Ther 10:1717–1728. doi:10.1517/14712598.2010.534079

56. Badylak SF, Taylor D, Uygun K (2011) Whole-organ tissue engineering: decellularization and recellularization of three-dimensional matrix scaffolds. Annu Rev Biomed Eng 13:27–53. doi:10.1146/annurev-bioeng-071910-124743

57. Moraes C, Mehta G, Lesher-Perez SC, Takayama S (2012) Organs-on-a-chip: a focus on compartmentalized microdevices. Ann Biomed Eng 40:1211–1227. doi:10.1007/s10439-011-0455-6

58. Powers MJ, Domansky K, Kaazempur-Mofrad MR, Kalezi A, Capitano A, Upadhyaya A, Kurzawski P, Wack KE, Stolz DB, Kamm R, Griffith LG (2002) A microfabricated array bioreactor for perfused 3D liver culture. Biotechnol Bioeng 78:257–269

59. Powers MJ, Janigian DM, Wack KE, Baker CS, Beer Stolz D, Griffith LG (2002) Functional behavior of primary rat liver cells in a three-dimensional perfused microarray bioreactor. Tissue Eng 8:499–513. doi:10.1089/107632702760184745

60. Shin M, Matsuda K, Ishii O, Terai H, Kaazempur-Mofrad M, Borenstein J, Detmar M, Vacanti JP (2004) Endothelialized networks with a vascular geometry in microfabricated poly(dimethyl siloxane). Biomed Microdevices 6:269–278. doi:10.1023/B:BMMD.0000048559.29932.27

61. Huh D, Fujioka H, Tung YC, Futai N, Paine R 3rd, Grotberg JB, Takayama S (2007) Acoustically detectable cellular-level lung injury induced by fluid mechanical stresses in microfluidic airway systems. Proc Natl Acad Sci USA 104:18886–18891. doi:10.1073/pnas.0610868104

62. Lam MT, Huang YC, Birla RK, Takayama S (2009) Microfeature guided skeletal muscle tissue engineering for highly organized 3-dimensional free-standing constructs. Biomaterials 30:1150–1155. doi:10.1016/j.biomaterials.2008.11.014

63. Huh D, Matthews BD, Mammoto A, Montoya-Zavala M, Hsin HY, Ingber DE (2010) Reconstituting organ-level lung functions on a chip. Science 328:1662–1668. doi:10.1126/science.1188302

64. Mao JJ, Vunjak-Novakovic G, Mikos AG, Atala A (eds) (2008) Translational approaches in tissue engineering and regenerative medicine. Artech House, Boston

65. Hutmacher DW, Sittinger M, Risbud MV (2004) Scaffold-based tissue engineering: rationale for computer-aided design and solid free-form fabrication systems. Trends Biotechnol 22:354–362. doi:10.1016/j.tibtech.2004.05.005

66. Huang Z-M, Zhang YZ, Kotaki M, Ramakrishna S (2003) A review on polymer nanofibers by electrospinning and their applications in nanocomposites. Compos Sci Technol 63:2223–2253. doi:10.1016/s0266-3538(03)00178-7

67. Quadrani P, Pasini A, Mattiolli-Belmonte M, Zannoni C, Tampieri A, Landi E, Giantomassi F, Natali D, Casali F, Biagini G, Tomei-Minardi A (2005) High-resolution 3D scaffold model for engineered tissue fabrication using a rapid prototyping technique. Med Biol Eng Comput 43:196–199

68. Erkizia G (2009) Modelling the microstructural degradation of scaffolds used in bone regeneration. University of Navarra, Spain

69. Sengers BG, Taylor M, Please CP, Oreffo RO (2007) Computational modelling of cell spreading and tissue regeneration in porous scaffolds. Biomaterials 28:1926–1940. doi:10.1016/j.biomaterials.2006.12.008

70. Bhardwaj N, Kundu SC (2010) Electrospinning: a fascinating fiber fabrication technique. Biotechnol Adv 28:325–347. doi:10.1016/j.biotechadv.2010.01.004
71. Erkizia G, Rainer A, de Juan-Pardo EM, Aldazabal J (2010) Computer simulation of scaffold degradation. Paper presented at Bio-Coat 2010, Zaragoza, Spain, June 24, 2010
72. Stylianopoulos T, Bashur CA, Goldstein AS, Guelcher SA, Barocas VH (2008) Computational predictions of the tensile properties of electrospun fibre meshes: effect of fibre diameter and fibre orientation. J Mech Behav Biomed Mater 1:326–335. doi:10.1016/j.jmbbm.2008.01.003
73. Hosseini SA, Tafreshi HV (2010) 3-D simulation of particle filtration in electrospun nanofibrous filters. Powder Technol 201:153–160. doi:10.1016/j.powtec.2010.03.020
74. Kowalewski TA, Blonski S, Barral S (2005) Experiments and modelling of electrospinning process. Bull Pol Acad Sci 53:385–394
75. Xu L, Wu Y, Nawaz Y (2011) Numerical study of magnetic electrospinning processes. Comput Math Appl 61:2116–2119. doi:10.1016/j.camwa.2010.08.085
76. Genovese J, Spadaccio C, Rainer A, Covino E (2011) Electrospun nanocomposites and stem cells in cardiac tissue engineering. In: Boccaccini AR, Harding SE (eds) Myocardial tissue engineering. Studies in mechanobiology, tissue engineering and biomaterials, vol 6. Springer, Berlin–Heidelberg
77. Sun W, Starly B, Nam J, Darling A (2005) Bio-CAD modeling and its applications in computer-aided tissue engineering. Comput Aided Des 37:1097–1114. doi:10.1016/j.cad.2005.02.002
78. Wei X, Xia Z, Wong S-C, Baji A (2009) Modelling of mechanical properties of electrospun nanofibre network. Int J Exp Comput Biomech 1:45–57. doi:10.1504/ijecb.2009.022858
79. Cioffi M, Boschetti F, Raimondi MT, Dubini G (2006) Modeling evaluation of the fluid-dynamic microenvironment in tissue-engineered constructs: a micro-CT based model. Biotechnol Bioeng 93:500–510. doi:10.1002/bit.20740
80. Sadir S, Öchsner A, Kadir MRA, Harun MN (2011) Simulation of direct perfusion through 3D cellular scaffolds with different porosity. Int Proc Chem Biol Environ Eng 5:123–126
81. Shin Y, Han S, Jeon JS, Yamamoto K, Zervantonakis IK, Sudo R, Kamm RD, Chung S (2012) Microfluidic assay for simultaneous culture of multiple cell types on surfaces or within hydrogels. Nat Protoc 7:1247–1259. doi:10.1038/nprot.2012.051
82. Lemon G, Howard D, Tomlinson MJ, Buttery LD, Rose FR, Waters SL, King JR (2009) Mathematical modelling of tissue-engineered angiogenesis. Math Biosci 221:101–120. doi:10.1016/j.mbs.2009.07.003
83. Erkizia G, Rainer A, de Juan-Pardo EM, Aldazabal J (2010) Computer simulation of scaffold degradation. J Phys Conf Ser 252:012004. doi:10.1088/1742-6596/252/1/012004
84. Erkizia G, de Juan-Pardo E, Kim G-M, Aldazabal J (2011) Computer simulation of manufacture, degradation and drug release of electrospun fibres. In: Fernandes PR, Bártolo PJ, Folgado J et al (eds) Proc 2nd intern conf tissue eng 2011. IST Press, Lisbon, pp 83–88
85. Chen Y, Zhou S, Li Q (2011) Mathematical modeling of degradation for bulk-erosive polymers: applications in tissue engineering scaffolds and drug delivery systems. Acta Biomater 7:1140–1149. doi:10.1016/j.actbio.2010.09.038
86. Erkizia G, de Juan-Pardo EM, Kim G-M, Estella-Hermoso de Mendoza A, Garbayo E, Aldazabal J (2011) Computer simulation of PLGA micro/nano particles degradation. Paper presented at Euro BioMat 2011, Jena, Germany, April 13–14, 2011
87. Guy RH, Hadgraft J (1981) Calculations of drug release rates from cylinders. Int J Pharm 8:159–165. doi:10.1016/0378-5173(81)90093-4
88. Guy RH, Hadgraft J, Kellaway IW, Taylor M (1982) Calculations of drug release rates from particles. Int J Pharm 11:199–207. doi:10.1016/0378-5173(82)90038-2
89. Erkizia G (2012) Computer simulation of drug delivery and degradation of scaffolds. PhD dissertation. University of Navarra, Spain

Photocrosslinkable Materials for the Fabrication of Tissue-Engineered Constructs by Stereolithography

Rúben F. Pereira and Paulo J. Bártolo

Abstract Stereolithography is an additive technique that produces three-dimensional (3D) solid objects using a multi-layer procedure through the selective photo-initiated curing reaction of a liquid photosensitive material. Stereolithographic processes have been widely employed in Tissue Engineering for the fabrication of temporary constructs, using natural and synthetic polymers, and polymer-ceramic composites. These processes allow the fabrication of complex structures with a high accuracy and precision at physiological temperatures, incorporating cells and growth factors without significant damage or denaturation. Despite recent advances on the development of novel biomaterials and biocompatible crosslinking agents, the main limitation of these techniques are the lack number of available photocrosslinkable materials, exhibiting appropriate biocompatibility and biodegradability. This chapter gives an overview of the current state-of-art of materials and stereolithographic techniques to produce constructs for tissue regeneration, outlining challenges for future research.

1 Introduction

Tissue engineering is recognized as a promising field to overcome some of the limitations of existing clinical treatments for the repair of damaged and dysfunctional tissues or organs, such as shortage of donors, chronic rejection or transmission of diseases. This interdisciplinary field involves principles from biological sciences and engineering for the development of biological substitutes to restore, maintain, or improve tissue function [9, 11, 15]. Despite the recent advances on the interaction between living cells and materials [32, 36, 112] allowed the development of functional scaffolds to support cell activity and potentially promote the repair of different tissues like skin [21, 84], bone [51, 110] or cartilage [47, 104], the development of cost-effective approaches for the regeneration of damaged tissues remains a great challenge.

R.F. Pereira · P.J. Bártolo (✉)
Centre for Rapid and Sustainable Product Development (CDRsp), Polytechnic Institute of Leiria, Leiria, Portugal
e-mail: paulo.bartolo@ipleiria.pt

P.R. Fernandes, P.J. Bártolo (eds.), *Tissue Engineering*,
Computational Methods in Applied Sciences 31, DOI 10.1007/978-94-007-7073-7_8,
© Springer Science+Business Media Dordrecht 2014

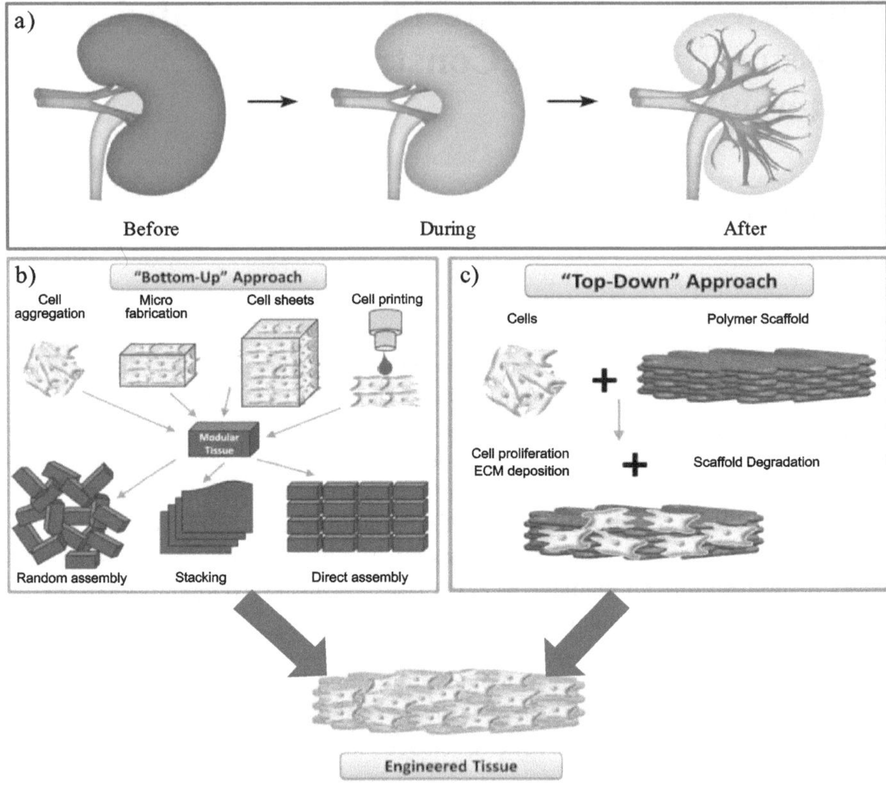

Fig. 1 Representative image of a kidney at different stages of the decellularization process (**a**). Bottom up (**b**) and top-down (**c**) approaches for tissue engineering (adapted from [75])

Decellularized tissue matrices gained increasing attention as a template for organ regeneration. These matrices, shown in Fig. 1a, were obtained from a donor and its cellular components removed, this way avoiding the risk of rejection and maintaining the 3D structure of the extracellular matrix (ECM) as a scaffold for organ regeneration [78, 88]. Currently, two fundamental strategies are considered for the development of biological substitutes for damaged tissues, namely the bottom-up (Fig. 1b) and the top-down (Fig. 1c) approaches [15, 75].

The bottom-up approach has emerged as a new method for the development of 3D biomimetic substitutes exploring the self-ability of cells to synthesize their own ECM without the need of supporting materials [15, 69, 73, 88]. Complex structures can be obtained through this approach by assembling modular tissues produced by different techniques, such as self-assembled aggregation, microfabrication of cell-laden hydrogels or direct printing [25, 75]. The top-down approach, commonly used one, is based on the use of porous and biodegradable matrices (scaffolds) to support cell attachment, proliferation and differentiation, guiding the formation of new tissue in an organized way [14, 15]. This approach involves the fabrication

Table 1 Biological, physical and mechanical requirements of scaffolds [1, 8, 14, 15]

Biological requisites	
Biocompatibility	Scaffold must be non-toxic and interact with biological tissues without inducing adverse responses
Biodegradability	Scaffold material should be gradually degraded in non-toxic products with appropriated molecular weights to allow the clearance from the human body
Degradation rate	The degradation rate should be adjustable and match the regeneration rate of the new tissue
Porosity	Scaffold must exhibit adequate pore size and interconnected pores. These properties are fundamental to promote an efficient cell seeding, nutrient and waste exchange, vascularization and tissue in-growth
Bioactivity	Scaffolds should be able to stimulate the attachment, proliferation and differentiation of the seeded cells, guiding the growth of the new tissue. The constructs should also be able to incorporate and deliver drugs and growth factors according to specific release profiles
Mechanical and physical requisites	
Mechanical strength	Scaffolds must present adequate strength and stiffness to support stresses in the host tissue environment. Mechanical properties should be similar to those in the native tissue, providing a temporary support to the tissue formation. During regeneration, scaffolds gradually transfer the mechanical loads and stresses to the new tissue
Surface finish	The surface chemistry of scaffolds should promote an optimal biomechanical coupling between the scaffold and the tissue, promoting cell attachment, differentiation and proliferation
Sterilization	Scaffolds must be easily sterilized using thermal, chemical or radiation processes, without degradation or modification of the material properties

of 3D biocompatible scaffolds and the manipulation of living cells and signalling molecules (e.g. growth factors), as well the *in vitro* culture of the cellular tissue-engineered constructs within bioreactors to promote the growing of clinically relevant healthy tissues. Scaffolds, from either natural or synthetic materials, play an important role on tissue regeneration, mimicking the function of the natural EMC of the human body. These structures act as a temporary support for the seeded autologous or allogeneic cells proliferation, differentiation, and synthesizing their own ECM [14, 15, 69]. Scaffolds need to successfully satisfy several requirements, as indicated in Table 1.

Several techniques can be used to produce scaffolds for tissue engineering applications, which can be classified as non-additive and additive biomanufacturing techniques.

Conventional techniques like solvent casting, freeze-drying, phase separation, gas foaming, melt molding and particle-leaching, are used to produce 3D scaffolds with relative control over the micro- and macro-scale features [41, 46, 77, 95, 106, 108]. However, these techniques present several limitations, such as the lack of control over the pore size and interconnectivity, porosity and pore spatial distribution [1, 15, 82, 109], leading to an inadequate vascularization and heterogeneous distribution of cells, promoting a non-uniform tissue growth [68]. In addition, these techniques usually employ toxic organic solvents, which prevent the incorporation of cells and other biological molecules during fabrication [15, 82].

Biomanufacturing represents a group of non-conventional fabrication techniques for the production of biological constructs for tissue engineering applications through the use of additive technologies, biodegradable and biocompatible materials, cells and growth factors [6, 7]. Additive biomanufacturing techniques produce complex 3D scaffolds in a layer-by-layer pattern from a CAD model, providing precise control over the pore size, porosity and pore interconnectivity [8, 15, 18, 82]. Several techniques, such as vat photopolymerization or stereolithographic processes, powder bed fusion processes, extrusion-based processes and inkjet processes have been developed, processing a wide range of materials, with a high level of automation and reproducibility [69]. Among these techniques, the vat photopolymerization processes are widely used for the production of scaffolds both containing or not encapsulated cells and growth factors, due to the ability to induce curing at physiological temperatures with a high accuracy, precision and resolution. Stereolithographic processes and different materials have been successfully used to produce tissue-engineered constructs. These materials are described in this chapter, highlighting different photofabrication approaches and applications.

2 Stereolithography

Stereolithography produces 3D solid objects in a multi-layer procedure through the selective photo-initiated curing reaction of a liquid photosensitive material containing a low-molecular weight pre-polymer, additives and photo-initiators [8, 15, 17, 65, 74]. The curing reaction is induced by a light source like ultraviolet (UV), infrared (IR) or visible light, supplying the necessary energy to bond a large number of small molecules, forming a highly cross-linked polymer [13, 15]. Radical polymerization is the most commonly used method to allow the photopolymerization, involving the generation of reactive species (free radicals) by the interaction with the incident light [26]. These species induce a curing reaction forming an insoluble and cross-linked 3D network. During this process, the liquid polymeric solution increases its viscosity as a result of the gelation, forming an elastic sol-gel structure. The sol fraction decreases and the polymer becomes more viscous, due to an increase in the number of cross-links between the polymeric chains. As the

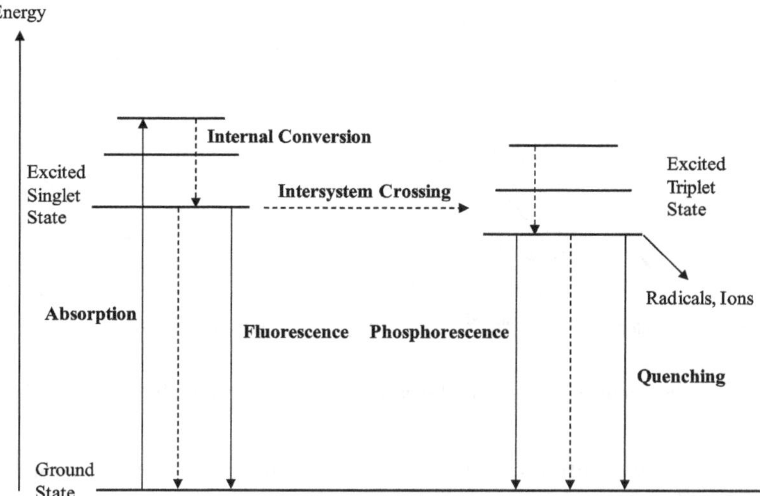

Fig. 2 Jablonski energy diagram

reaction proceeds, the material becomes more cross-linked, its molecular weight increases and a glassy solid material is formed [13]. The curing reaction is highly dependent on the light intensity, temperature, irradiation time, and photo-initiator concentration [13]. Either a single-photon polymerization or a two-photon polymerization (2PP) can be used to induce the curing reaction. The chemical principle of these two processes is similar, though they differ in the number of absorbed photons required to induce the polymerization process [13, 82]. When a molecule absorbs light, the electrons are set into motion by the oscillating electric field, which is promoted from the highest occupied molecular orbital to an unoccupied molecular orbital with the formation of an excited singlet state molecule. However, this excited molecule is a short living species (less than 10^{-8} s), which disappears by various competitive processes dissipating the excited energy. The absorption of light by a molecule and the subsequent evolution of its excited states can be observed in Fig. 2 through the Jablonski energy diagram.

Two processes can be identified, the photophysical and the photochemical ones, as follows:

- Photophysical processes:

  – Radiative
  – Non-radiative

- Photochemical processes.

Radiative mechanisms involve both the absorption of a photon or more by a molecule in its ground state (S_0) and the emission of energy from an electronically excited state, by either fluorescence (de-excitation of an excited state with the same spin multiplicity as the ground state) or phosphorescence (de-excitation of

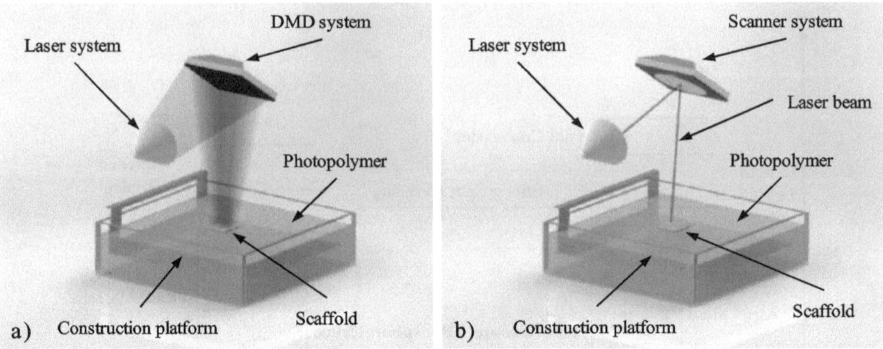

Fig. 3 Stereolithographic processes: mask-based (**a**) and laser writing (**b**) methods

an excited state with different spin multiplicity as the ground state). Non-radiative processes include internal conversion (IC) and intersystem crossing (ISC), which occurs among different spin multiplicity states creating excited triplet states (T_1). The photochemical processes imply the transformation of the starting molecule through cleavage processes, electron transfer reactions, hydrogen abstraction, etc. Most photochemical reactions occur only via excited triplet states, which are longer live species (greater than 10^{-6} s). Singlet or triplet states are electronic states where the molecule has either paired electrons or unpaired electrons, respectively.

Stereolithographic processes usually employ two distinct methods of irradiation: the mask-based method (Fig. 3a) and the direct or laser writing method (Fig. 3b) [12].

In the mask-based method, an image is transferred to a liquid polymer by irradiation through a patterned mask, which contains transparent zones corresponding to the sections of the model to be built [8]. This process enables the curing of one entire layer in just one irradiation step, this way reducing the fabrication time and avoiding undesirable polymerizations as a result of the low-density flux of light over the polymer surface [15, 71, 85]. However, the mask-based approach requires the generation of a great number of masks with precise alignments, which can be done by using Liquid Crystal Display (LCD) panels and Digital Micromirror Devices (DMD's) as dynamic pattern generators [13, 85].

The direct or laser writing method is the most commonly used one, involving the use of a focused laser beam to selectively irradiate and solidify the liquid photopolymer [8]. In this case, the stereolithography apparatus consists of a computer, a vat containing a photosensitive liquid polymer, a moveable platform in which the model is built, a laser to irradiate and cure the photosensitive resin, and a dynamic mirror system to guide and project the laser beam over the polymer surface. After the curing of the first layer, the platform dips into the polymer vat and leaves a thin film of liquid polymer in the surface of the first layer, which is then irradiated to produce the second layer [15, 16]. Once the depth of curing is larger than the resin layer (Fig. 4), a good adhesion between the different layers of the model is ensured [71].

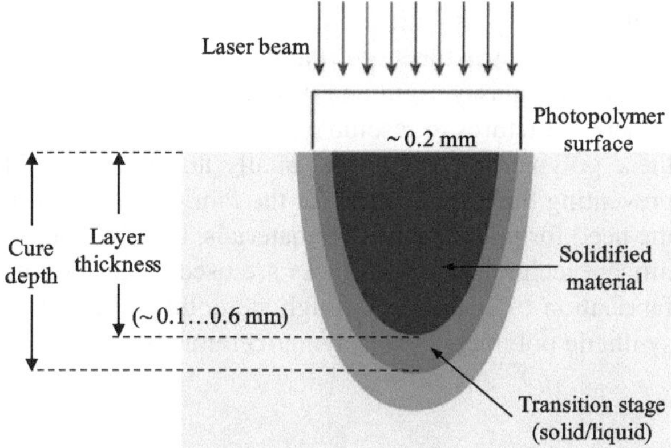

Fig. 4 Irradiation phenomena

Conventional stereolithography has been successfully applied for the fabrication of tissue-engineered constructs using several natural and synthetic materials [58, 68, 115]. However, the fabrication of porous 3D constructs with an interconnected micro-architecture is limited by the resolution of the system [27]. Microstereolithography is a process that evolved from conventional stereolithography, allowing the fabrication of complex 3D constructs with a micro-scale resolution of about 200 nm [27, 55, 71]. In this process, the laser beam is more precisely focused, reducing the spot size to a few micrometers in diameter, this way enhancing the resolution of the system [13, 56]. Today, there is a great interest in the use of 2PP processes for the fabrication of various devices, such as microneedles, sensors and scaffolds for different biological and biomedical applications [39, 48, 53]. These processes are able to produce 3D structures with submicron resolution, enabling an ultra-fast fabrication process at greater depth [8]. However, 2PP systems are very expensive, operating with a single material type that prevents the fabrication of multimaterial constructs [85]. These equipments usually employ a femtosecond titanium:sapphire laser (short pulse width and high peak power) without photo-masks, operating at approximately 800 nm wavelength to induce the polymerization [53, 74, 82]. A great variety of natural and synthetic photosensitive materials can be used for the 2PP technique, like acrylate-based polymer, zirconium sol-gels, organically modified ceramic materials, aliphatic polyesters and gelatin [52, 74, 79, 105].

Despite these processes enable to produce complex 3D scaffolds with pre-defined micro/nanoscale architectures, the major limitation of stereolithographic processes for tissue engineering applications consists on the lack of available photocurable, biocompatible and biodegradable materials.

3 Materials for Stereolithography

The first polymeric systems developed for stereolithography were based on low-molecular weight polyacrylate or epoxy macromers, which present a rapid cure and enable an easy modification at the ester functionality [13, 44, 71, 91]. However, the obtained structures are scarcely applied on tissue engineering as they are predominantly glassy, rigid and brittle, preventing the fabrication of flexible and elastomeric structures to resemble the properties of human tissues [13, 58]. In addition, these polymeric systems are usually not biocompatible or biodegradable, thereby preventing their application for the fabrication of scaffolds [35, 44, 91]. To address the need for photocurable biomaterials, both biocompatible and biodegradable, significant technological advances are used to develop novel polymeric systems. The fabrication of scaffolds through stereolithography involves the use of natural and synthetic polymers, and polymer/ceramic blends.

3.1 Polymers

Polymeric materials are the most commonly used materials for biomedical applications, due to the wide range of its properties, easy processing and versatility. Both natural and synthetic polymers can be modified to allow the processing through stereolithography, without affecting or even improving the interaction with living cells.

Biocompatible hydrogels, based on either natural or synthetic polymers, represent a relevant group of materials widely employed for several biomedical applications, including tissue engineering [97], wound dressings [84], controlled drug delivery [113] and cell encapsulation [103]. Hydrogels are tridimensional hydrophilic networks with the ability to absorb and retain large amounts of water without dissolution [84], due to the establishment of physical (reversible) or chemical (irreversible) bonds between the polymeric chains [43, 69, 98, 100]. These are attractive materials for tissue engineering applications due to its excellent biocompatibility, biodegradability, elasticity, smoothness and compositional similarities regarding the ECM of the human body [43, 98, 101]. In addition, some hydrogels can be photopolymerized using *in vitro* and *in vivo* conditions in the presence of cells and photoinitiators [13, 63, 100, 111], which can potentially improve its use for the *in situ* regeneration of damaged tissues. The high water content of the hydrogels makes them useful carriers for the transport and delivery of fragile molecules (e.g. proteins, drugs or cells), providing a 3D environment similar to the one in human tissues, protecting these molecules from denaturation or degradation [69, 98, 101]. It is possible to manipulate the diffusion and transport of biological materials by changing both the density of cross-links and the pore size of the gel network. The control over the cross-links density also enables to tailor different properties, such as its swelling behavior, degradation rate, mechanical properties, pore size and permeability [50, 69].

Hydrogels used in stereolithography comprise natural polymers (e.g. alginate, chitosan, hyaluronic acid, gelatin), synthetic polymers (e.g. poly(ethyleneglycol) (PEG), propylene fumarate (PPF), poly(ε-caprolactone) (PCL)) and a combination of both [13, 59, 100, 101]. Synthetic and natural hydrogels are usually modified using photoreactive and crosslinkable groups, such as acrylates and methacrylates, to enable their processing by stereolithographic processes [4, 69, 71, 111].

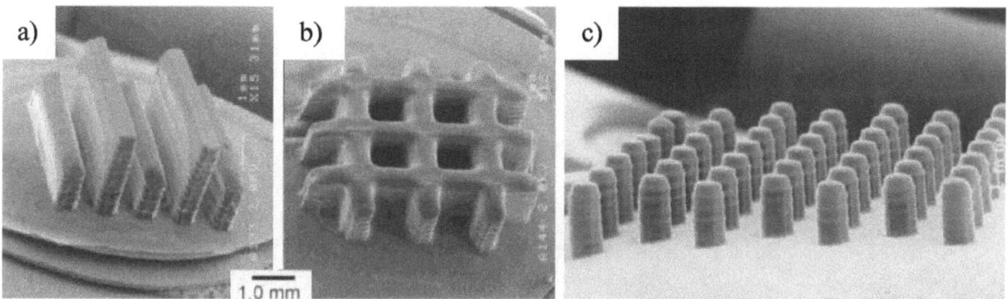

Fig. 5 Scanning electron microscopy (SEM) images of microbanks (**a**), microwells (**b**) and microneedle-array (**c**) built by stereolithography using the CL and TMC oligomers [66]

3.1.1 Synthetic Polymers and Hydrogels

The interest on synthetic polymers concerns good and adjustable physical, chemical and mechanical properties, easy processing into a wide range of shapes and large-scale production. On the other hand, their main drawback regard its limited biocompatibility, poor interaction with living cells, and in some cases the toxicity of the degradation products [87, 96]. The surface of synthetic polymers can be modified through different approaches, such as plasma treatment, polymer coating, chemical modification, peptide immobilization and photochemical modifications, to improve cell interactions or provide specific interactions with different cell types [40, 102].

In stereolithography, the most used biodegradable macromers are based on functionalized oligomers containing hydrolyzable ester- or carbonate linkages in the main chain [71]. Examples include PPF [56], PCL [35], poly(D,L-lactide) (PDLLA) [70] and poly(trimethylene carbonate) (PTMC) [89]. Usually, these polymers are mixed with reactive and non-reactive diluents, such as diethyl fumarate (DEF), to control the viscosity and the degree of cross-linking, allowing the fabrication of constructs with adequate mechanical properties [35, 50, 58, 71].

Matsuda et al. [67] reported the preparation of photocurable liquid biodegradable copolymers through the ring-opening copolymerization of ε-caprolactone (CL) and trimethylene carbonate (TMC), using polyol as initiator and tin(II) 2-ethylhexanoate as a catalyst. The copolymers were subsequently derivated at the hydroxyl end with a photodimerizable coumarin group. Results showed that higher coumarin functionality and UV light intensity, and a reduced layer thickness of the liquid film precursor increases the photocuring reaction. The same oligomers were used by Matsuda and Mizutani [66] to produce photocurable copolymers, using trimethylene glycol or PEG as initiator and an acrylate group (acryloyl chloride) to end-functionalize the oligomers. Different structures were produced using the photocurable copolymers through stereolithography, as shown in Fig. 5.

PPF, an unsaturated linear polyester, has been used in stereolithography due to its ability to be cross-linked through the carbon-carbon double bonds, presenting excellent mechanical properties [54, 87]. The subunits of PPF can be crosslinked by using different agents, such as DEF, methyl methacrylate and N-vinylpyrrolidone [54]. In addition, PPF also undergoes degradation into biocompatible and non-toxic

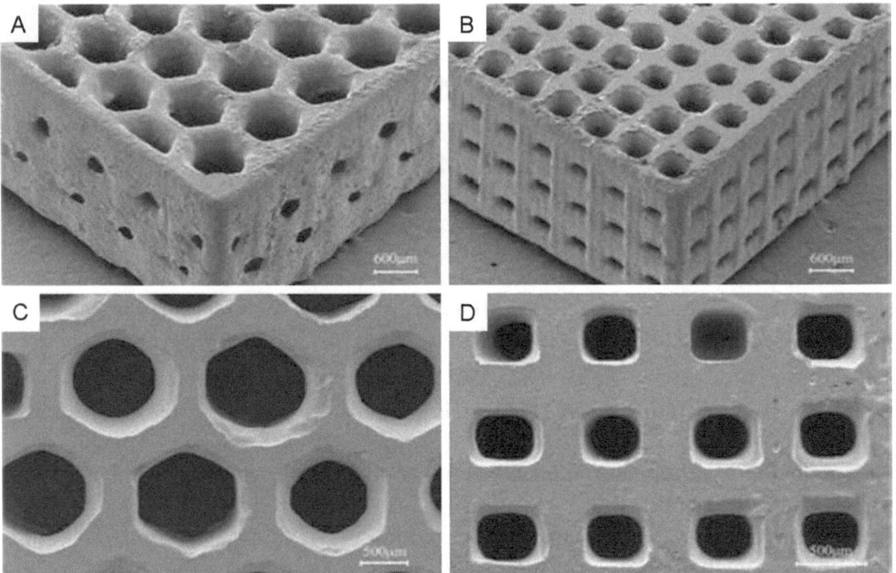

Fig. 6 SEM images of PPF scaffolds, with different pores shapes (hexagon (**A**, **C**) and square (**B**, **D**) pores) and pore sizes (600 μm for hexagon and 508 μm for square) [58]

fumaric acid and propylene glycol products by simple hydrolysis of the ester bonds [57, 58, 87].

Lee et al. [58] produced 3D scaffolds for tissue engineering using a UV curable polymer solution, consisting of PPF, DEF as a solvent and bisacrylphosphrine oxide (BAPO) as a photoinitiator. The composition of the photocurable solution and the laser parameters were optimized and scaffolds with different pore sizes, pore shapes and porosities were produced (Fig. 6). Similarly, Lee et al. [57] used a microstereolithography system to produce PPF scaffolds with control over the pore size, porosity, interconnectivity and pore distribution. After 1 week of *in vitro* culture, fibroblasts showed good adhesion and spreading on both bottom and side construct walls.

However, synthetic polymers like PPF are hydrophobic and low bioactive materials. To solve these limitations, Lan et al. [54] coated PPF scaffolds produced by microstereolithography with accelerated biomimetic apatite and arginini-glycine-aspartic acid peptide coating. Similarly, Shin et al. [94] used three different peptides, Arg–Gly–Asp (RGD), cyclo RGD and a mixture of RGD-KRSR (lysine–arginine–serine–arginine), to improve the surface properties of PPF/DEF scaffolds for bone tissue engineering applications. The modified scaffolds were seeded with MC3T3-E1 pre-osteoblasts, and the effect of each peptide on the cell adhesion, proliferation and differentiation was evaluated. Results showed that the peptide modification enhanced the adhesion and proliferation of MC3T3-E1 pre-osteoblasts, comparatively to the non-modified scaffolds.

Stereolithography has also been used to produce scaffolds for the delivery of growth factors. Lee et al. [56] produced 3D scaffolds containing bone morphogenetic protein-2 (BMP-2)-loaded poly(DL-lactic-coglycolic acid) (PLGA) microspheres (Fig. 7), by the polymerization of a suspension consisting of a PPF/DEF photopolymer and microspheres. In this work, scaffolds were also produced through a conventional process (particulate leaching/gas foaming) to evaluate the influence of the fabrication process on the scaffold performance. Results showed that scaffolds, produced by microstereolithography, provide a better environment for cell proliferation and differentiation. To evaluate the *in vivo* bone formation, scaffolds were implanted into a rat cranial defect. After 11 weeks of implantation, it was possible to observe a significant bone formation on the defect treated using the BMP-2-loaded scaffold, produced by microstereolithography (Fig. 7).

Thermoplastic aliphatic polyesters, such as PCL, poly(lactic acid) (PLA) and poly(glycolic acid) (PGA), represent another class of synthetic polymers extensively applied for the fabrication of tissue engineering scaffolds through stereolithography. The large number of existing aliphatic polyesters offers the possibility to prepare structures with distinct properties. For example, lactide-based precursors have been used to fabricate hard and rigid structures for both orthopedic and bone tissue applications, while the copolyester precursors are employed for the fabrication of flexible and elastomeric structures suitable for soft-tissue applications [92].

PCL is a biodegradable, biocompatible and semi-crystalline polymer FDA approved for various applications, such as sutures, wound dressings and stents [28, 83, 99]. This material presents a low melting point and its degradation kinetics, physical and mechanical properties can be easily adjusted by different approaches, including the (i) manipulation of the polymer molecular weight, (ii) the copolymer ratio, (iii) the blending with other polymers, and (iv) the incorporation of labile bonds into the backbone [35, 87].

Elomaa et al. [35] synthesized three-armed PCL oligomers by ring-opening polymerization of ε-caprolactone monomers. The photocrosslinkable PCL-based resin was end-functionalized with methacrylic anhydride, and subsequently employed to produce 3D porous scaffolds trough a mask stereolithographic system. The produced scaffolds exhibited porosity of 70.5 %, pore size in the range of 400–500 μm, and a high interconnectivity between pores without material shrinkage. NIH3T3 fibroblasts, cultured on photocrosslinked PCL networks, can be easily attached presenting uniform spreading.

Two-photon polymerization has been explored to produce scaffolds using PCL-based polymers. Claeyssens et al. [31] fabricated 3D structures composed of the biodegradable triblock copolymer poly(ε-caprolactone-co-trimethylenecarbonate)-b-poly(ethylene glycol)-b-poly(ε-caprolactoneco-trimethylenecarbonate), using 4,4′-bis(diethylamino) benzophenone as the photoinitiator. Constructs with different geometries were prepared with a resolution of 4 μm (Fig. 8). Fibroblasts, cultured onto spin-coated thin films after photopolymerization, remained viable and showed comparable cell attachment and division regarding cells cultured on glass surfaces (control), which indicates that the developed material do not affect cell proliferation. In a similar work, Koskela et al. [53] used the 2PP technique to produce

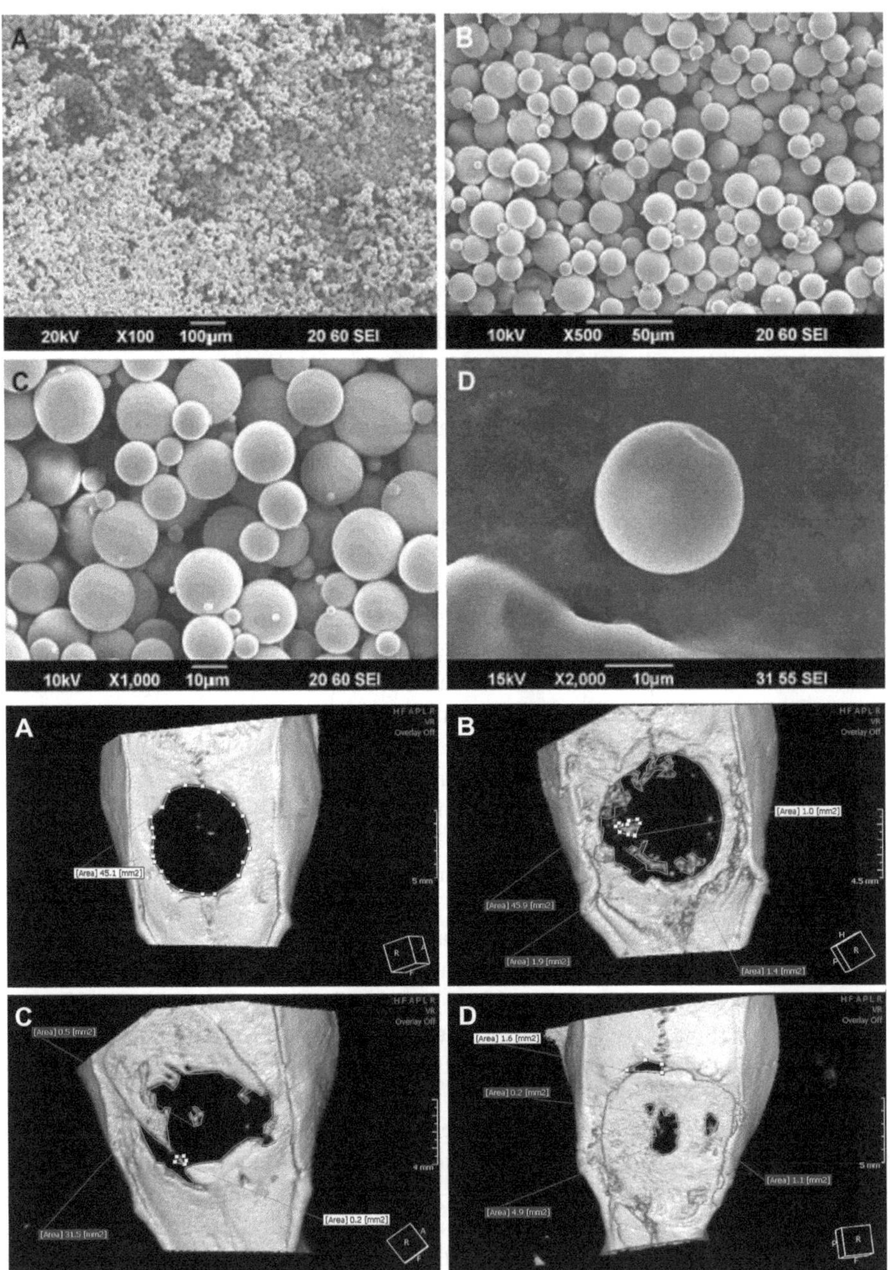

Fig. 7 *Left*: SEM images of the BMP-2-loaded microspheres. *Right*: Micro-CT images of rat cranial bone, at 11 weeks after implantation: (**A**) Negative control, (**B**) BMP-2-unloaded particulate leaching/gas foaming scaffold, (**C**) BMP-2-unloaded microstereolithography scaffold, (**D**) BMP-2-loaded microstereolithography scaffold [56]

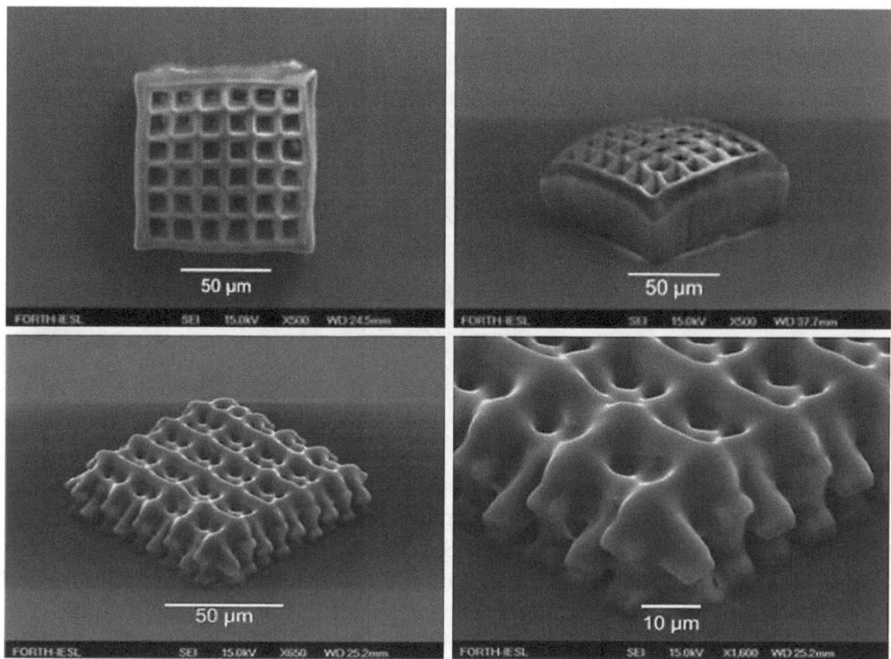

Fig. 8 SEM images of different 3D structures fabricated by two-photon polymerization [31]

microstructures, using methacrylated PCL-based oligomer (PCL-o) and Irgacure® 127 as UV photoinitiator. Live/dead staining analysis showed that hESC-derived neuronal cells, cultured on the PCL film for 7 days, were able to attach to the surface, though the material did not allow cell migration.

PLA is a biodegradable polymer available in three forms: L-PLA (PLLA), D-PLA (PDLA) and a racemic mixture of PDLLA [87]. The stereochemical structure of PLA can be modified by polymerizing a controlled mixture of L- or D-isomers, yielding amorphous or crystalline polymers [37]. PLA undergoes simple hydrolysis of the ester bond, and its degradation rate is highly dependent on the isomer ratio, the temperature of hydrolysis, as well the size and shape of the construct [37]. Recently, a photo-curable PDLLA-based material free of reactive diluents was developed, through functionalization with methacryloyl chloride [70]. This polymeric system was used for the fabrication of porous scaffolds with a gyroid architecture (Fig. 9), by using ethyl lactate as a non-reactive diluent. Pre-osteoblast cells, cultured on the scaffolds, showed good adhesion and proliferation. Jansen et al. [44] prepared biodegradable 3D porous scaffolds with a well-defined gyroid architecture (Fig. 9) and a porosity of 76 %, using photocross-linked networks based on fumaric acid monoethyl ester (FAME) end-functionalized PDLLA oligomers and N-vinyl-2-pyrrolidone, as a reactive diluent (PDLLA 3-FAME/NVP). Biological studies showed that mouse preosteoblast cells readily adhere and spread well onto disk-shaped polymeric networks. Koroleva et al. [52] used a photocurable and biodegrad-

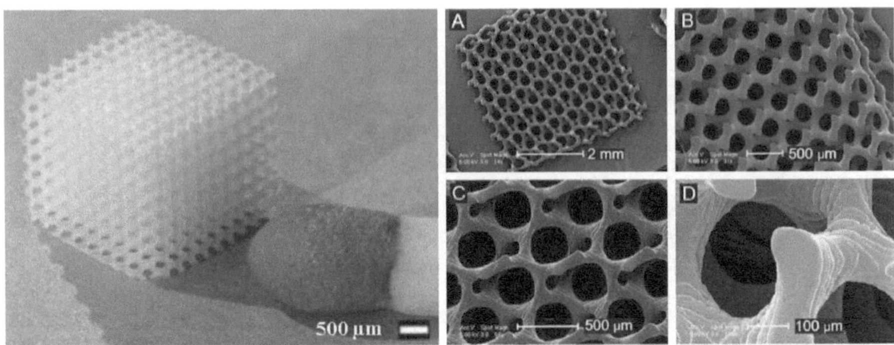

Fig. 9 *Left*: PDLLA scaffold built by stereolithography [70]. *Right*: SEM images of the PDLLA 3-FAME/NVP stereolithographic scaffold [44]

able PLA resin for the fabrication of 3D scaffolds. The potential of this polymeric material for neuronal tissue engineering applications was evaluated through the culture of rat primary Schwann cells and SH-SY5Y neuroblastoma cell line. Cells showed good adherence to the methacrylated PLA films, assuming spindle-like and flat cell morphologies when cultured on the 3D scaffolds. Results revealed the neurocompatibility of the developed constructs as well its ability to support cell proliferation.

Methacrylate end-functionalized PTMC macromers were used by Schüller-Ravoo et al. [89] to produce 3D constructs with a gyroid pore network. Before processing, the macromers were diluted using non-reactive propylene carbonate to decrease the viscosity and increase the processing temperature. The resulting network films exhibited high flexibility and elasticity, while the 3D porous scaffolds presented porosities in the range of 53–66 %. Meyer et al. [72] used the 2PP technique to produce 3D vessels with a branched tubular structure by, irradiating α, ω-polytetrahydrofuranether-diacrylate polymers. Tubular structures were obtained with a height of 160 μm, an inner diameter of 18 μm and a wall thickness of approximately 3 μm.

Synthetic hydrogels have also been processed through stereolithographic processes, such as poly(ethylene oxide) (PEO), poly(vinyl alcohol) (PVA), poly(butylene oxide) (PBO), poly(hydroxybutyrate) (PHB), polyacylamide, poly(hydroxypropyl methacrylamide) (PHPMA), poly(2-hydroxyethyl methacrylate) (PHEMA) and PEG [8].

PEG hydrogels are the most commonly used for conventional stereolithography [91], microstereolithography [63] and 2PP [80]. These materials exhibit high hydrophilicity, excellent biocompatibility, and can be functionalized with photoreactive end groups, such as acrylates or methacrylates, allowing the photopolymerization process [2]. Furthermore, PEG hydrogels can be susceptible to the hydrolytic degradation by the cleavage of the ester bonds, through either the introduction of proteolytically degradable peptide sequences into the backbone or by blending PEG with other biodegradable polymers [3, 24, 91]. Several works showed that PEG-based hydrogels can be modified with cell adhesive peptides, improving the cellular

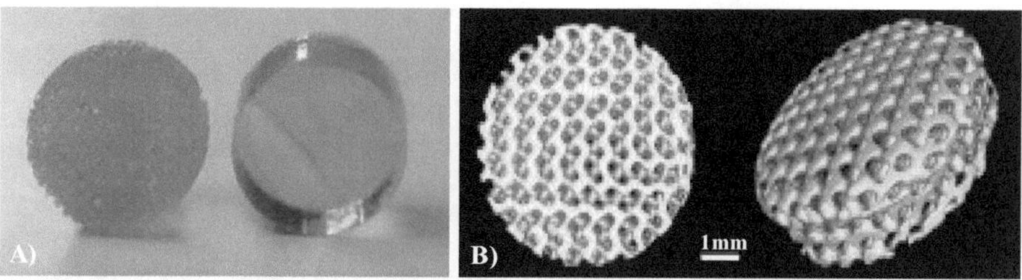

Fig. 10 (**A**) Porous (*left*) and solid (*right*) hydrogel structures built by stereolithography using methacrylate-functionalized poly(ethylene glycol)poly(D-Lactide), after several hours of extraction. (**B**) Micro-CT images of the porous constructs [91]

interaction, which can be processed by incorporating living cells at physiological conditions [24, 61–64, 115].

Seck et al. [91] produced porous and non-porous biodegradable hydrogel structures, using an aqueous photocurable polymer based on methacrylate-functionalized PEG/PDLLA macromers and Lucirin TPO-L as a visible light photo-initiator (Fig. 10A). Porous constructs were obtained with a gyroid pore network, 52 % of porosity and a fully interconnected pore network (Fig. 10B). Human mesenchymal stem cells, cultured on porous hydrogel structures, showed good adhesion and proliferation.

The fabrication of hydrogel scaffolds containing living cells and using stereolithographic processes was also tested. Bryant and Anseth [22] encapsulated chondrocytes into PEO hydrogels structures with a variable thickness, using an UV irradiation time of 10 minutes and a low light intensity ($\sim$10 mW/cm^2). The chondrocytes, encapsulated in the hydrogel structures and cultured *in vitro* during 6 weeks, remained viable and produced cartilaginous tissue. Lu et al. [63] used a dynamic masking system to produce scaffolds containing murine OP-9 marrow stromal cells. The cells were added to a polymeric system consisting of poly(ethylene glycol) diacrylate (PEGDA), dissolved into phosphate buffered saline and Irgacure 2959 as photo-initiator, and subsequently polymerized. After 24 hours of incubation, fluorescence microscopy analysis showed that cells maintained its viability. Using different fluorescently-labeled polystyrene microparticles, authors also showed the feasibility of the system to produce scaffolds with entrapped multiple biochemical factors presenting precise pre-designed and spatially-patterned layers (Fig. 11).

Lin et al. [61] incorporated living cells within PEGDA hydrogel scaffolds using a visible light-based projection stereolithography system. A commercial stereolithographic system, operating in a visible light mode (Hg illumination with UV barrier filter), was used to irradiate a monomer solution containing human adipose-derived stem cells, and lithium phenyl-2,4,6-trimethylbenzoylphosphinate as photoinitiator. After 7 days, it was possible to observe that cells maintained viability up to 90 %.

To reproduce the high complexity and heterogeneity of the human tissues, characterized by the presence of multiple ECM constituents and cells, it is critical to be able to produce 3D constructs containing heterogeneous layers, combining a variety

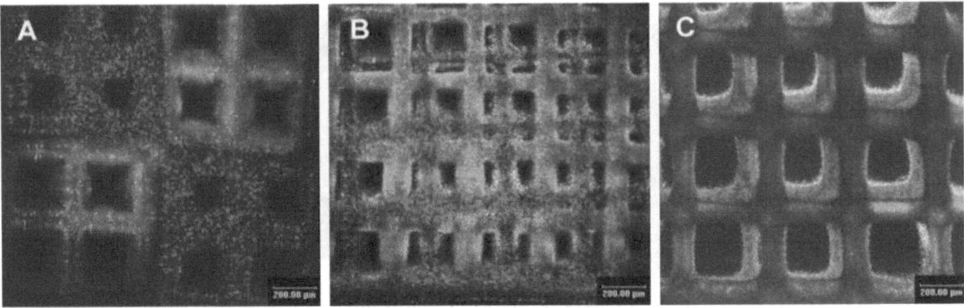

Fig. 11 Fluorescence confocal microscopy of PEGDA hydrogel scaffolds produced with pre-defined spatial-pattern in a single layer (**A**) and multi-layered scaffolds (**B, C**) containing either FITC or Cy5-labeled polystyrene particles [63]

of biomaterials and cells with precise spatial arrangement. Arcaute et al. [2–4] explored stereolithography for fabricating multi-material spatially controlled bioactive scaffolds. To accomplish multi-material fabrication, a mini-vat setup was designed, allowing for self-aligning X–Y registration during fabrication. The mini-vat setup allowed the construct to be easily removed and rinsed, and different photocrosslinkable solutions to be easily removed and added to the vat. Multi-material scaffolds were fabricated by including controlled concentrations of fluorescently labeled dextran, fluorescently labeled bioactive PEG or bioactive PEG in different regions of the scaffold (Fig. 12). Human dermal fibroblast cells were seeded on top of the fabricated scaffolds. Spatial control was successfully showed in features down to 500 μm.

Ovsianikov et al. [81] combined the 2PP technique and the laser-induced forward transfer (LIFT) process to produce 3D multicellular tissue constructs. The 2PP technique was employed for the fabrication of PEGDA scaffolds, which were subsequently seeded with vascular smooth muscle-like cells (within the outer scaffold area) and endothelial cells (into the inner scaffold area), using the LIFT process. To allow the fabrication of 3D constructs containing multiple hydrogel compositions and cell types with control over the spatial distribution of cells and bioactive molecules, Chan et al. [24] modified a conventional stereolithographic apparatus. These authors showed the production of PEGDA constructs with encapsulated/3T3 cells through the manual addition of individual layers of cell-containing photopolymer, preventing the cells settling to the bottom of the stereolithographic vat due to gravity.

Zorlutuna et al. [115] used stereolithography to produce spatially organized 3D co-culture of multiple cell types to investigate cell-cell interaction and the microenvironments of complex tissues. Two layer-constructs, using different cell types and hydrogels, were produced as shown in Fig. 13. The first layer was produced by polymerizing poly(ethylene glycol) methyl ether methacrylate (PEGMA3400) containing adipose-derived stem cells (ASCs), while the second layer contains primary hippocampus neurons (HNs) and skeletal muscle myoblast (MCs) cells encapsulated in oxidized methacrylic alginate and poly(ethylene glycol) methyl ether methacrylate 1100 (OMA-PEGMA1100).

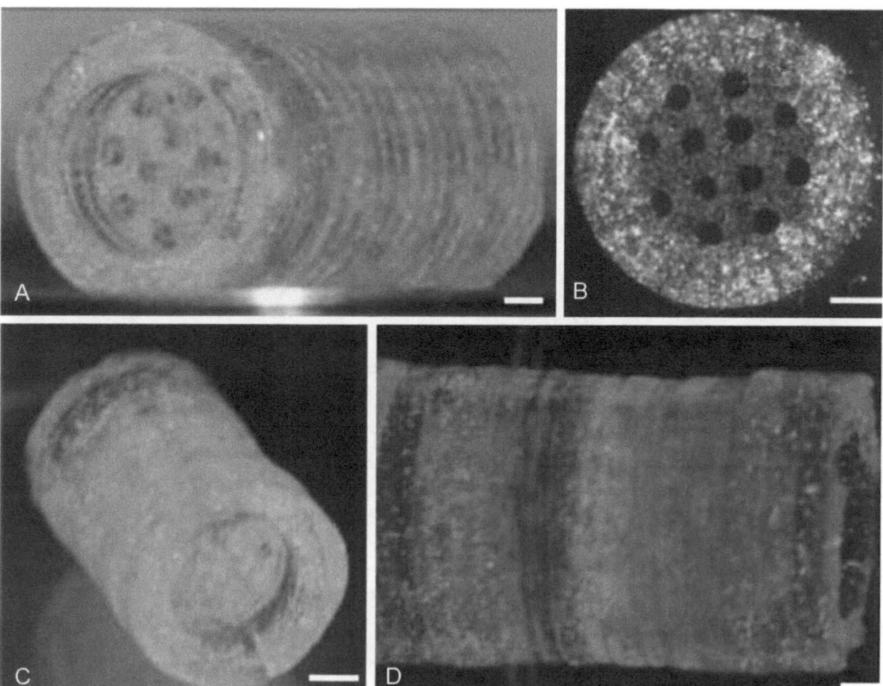

Fig. 12 Nerve guidance conduit produced using different colors of fluorescent particles in the PEG-based solution (the scale bar is 1 mm) [4]

3.1.2 Natural Polymers and Hydrogels

Recently, the use of natural polymers for biomedical applications has attracted an increase interest, due to its excellent properties, such as biodegradability, biocompatibility, low toxicity, availability, similar properties to the human tissues and inherent cellular interaction [42, 84]. When compared to synthetic polymers, these materials offer several advantages including biological signaling, cell adhesion and cell responsive degradation [87]. The main drawbacks of natural polymers regards the limited stability of its mechanical properties, low processing window and the risk of immune rejection [42, 86, 87, 96]. The use of these materials on stereolithography is still in its infancy, despite recent advances on the modification of natural polymers to allow its photo-crosslinking. Generally, natural polymers are modified by the introduction of methacrylate groups on the backbone to yield photopolymerizable materials. Examples include photocrosslinkable natural polymers like gelatin [76, 90], hyaluronic acid [5], alginate [45], chitosan [114] and silk fibroin [107]. These materials are explored in stereolithography manly to produce hydrogel scaffolds with and without encapsulated cells.

Gelatin is a natural polymer derived from collagen, one of the main constituents of ECM matrix, commonly used to produce scaffolds for tissue engineering, due

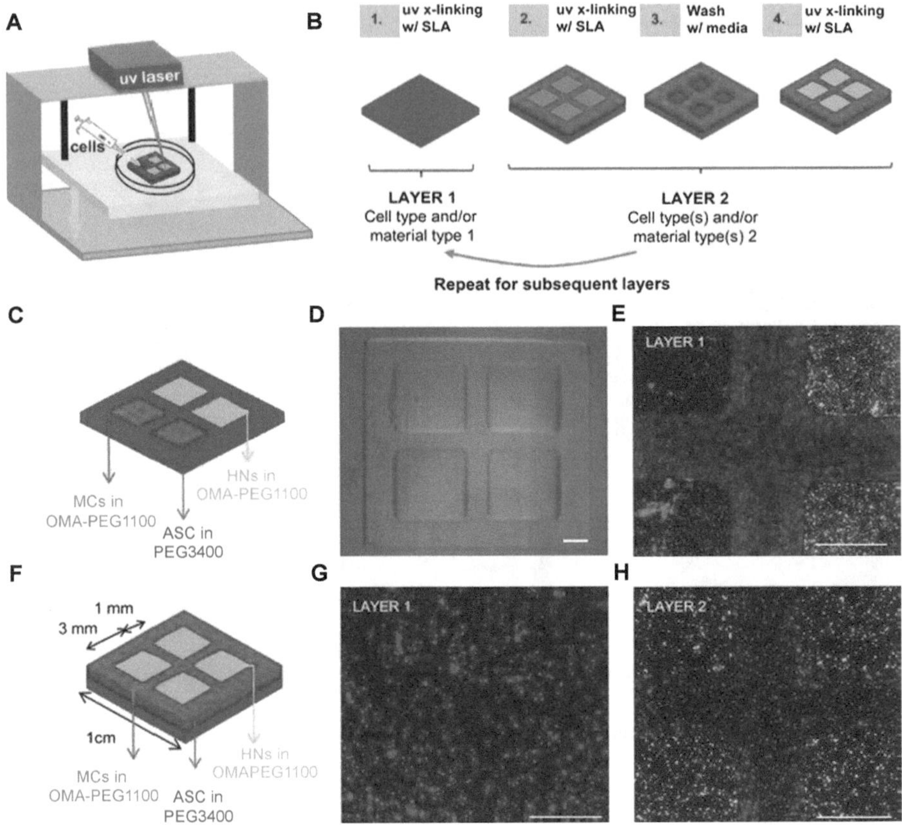

Fig. 13 Illustration of SLA process (**A**). Fabrication sequence (**B**). CAD models (**C, F**). Stereomicroscopy image of the produced hydrogel (**D**). Fluorescence microscopy images of the encapsulated MCs (*red*), HNs (*green*), and ASCs (*blue*) cells in different regions of the same layer (**E**); ASCs in the first layer (**G**) and HNs and MCs in the second layer (**H**). Scale bar represents 1 mm [115]

to its biodegradability and ability to provide good cell interaction and proliferation. Gauvin et al. [38] used a projection stereolithography system to produce scaffolds using gelatin methacrylate. Human umbilical vein endothelial cells, cultured on the porous scaffolds, exhibited good proliferation and maintained the endothelial phenotype. The 2PP technique was employed by Ovsianikov et al. [79] to produce 3D scaffolds using methacrylamide-modified gelatin (GelMOD), and Irgacure 2959 as photoinitiator (Fig. 14). After gelatin modification with the methacrylamide, it was observed that the *in vitro* degradation behavior of the polymer was not affected. The gelatin-based hydrogels showed ability to support the adhesion and proliferation of porcine mesenchymal stem cells, as well the capacity to induce the cellular differentiation into the anticipated lineage, upon applying osteogenic stimulation.

Basu et al. [19] prepared collagen (type I, II, IV) scaffolds with benzophenone dimer photoactivator using multiphoton (two- and three-photon excitation) poly-

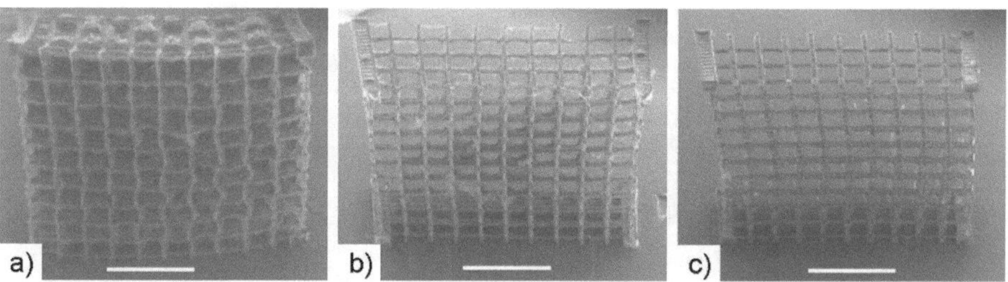

Fig. 14 Gelatin-based scaffolds built by 2PP process. Bar corresponds to 1 mm [79]

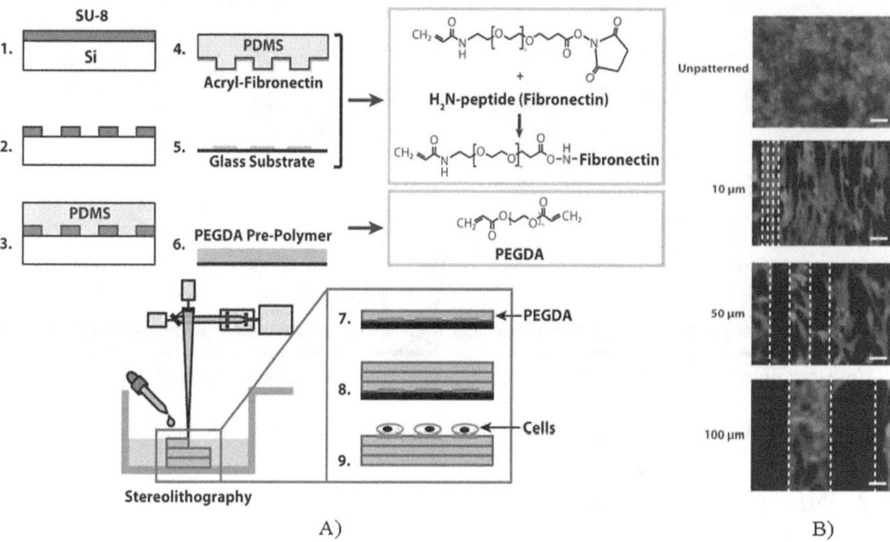

Fig. 15 (**A**) Fabrication procedure used to create patterns of acryl-fibronectin on the backbone of PEGDA hydrogels produced by stereolithography. (**B**) Fibroblasts aligned on the unpatterned and patterned hydrogels substrates [23]

merization. Scaffolds were crosslinked with the benzophenone dimer, and structures at sub-micrometer and micrometer scale were obtained. Results showed that the degradation rate of these structures can be tailored by changing the degree of cross-linking of collagen during fabrication. Primary human dermal fibroblasts cultured on the collagen structures showed good adhesion, so there is biocompatibility in the designed constructs. Chan et al. [23] developed a simple method for aligning cells on 3D hydrogels, by combining the micro-contact printing technique and stereolithography (Fig. 15). They modified fibronectin with acrylate groups, creating patterns of acryl-fibronectin on the backbone of PEGDA hydrogels produced by stereolithography, using a micro-contact printing technique. The cell alignment in the direction of the patterns created on the hydrogel substrates, was showed by the culture of the NIH/3T3 mouse embryonic fibroblasts.

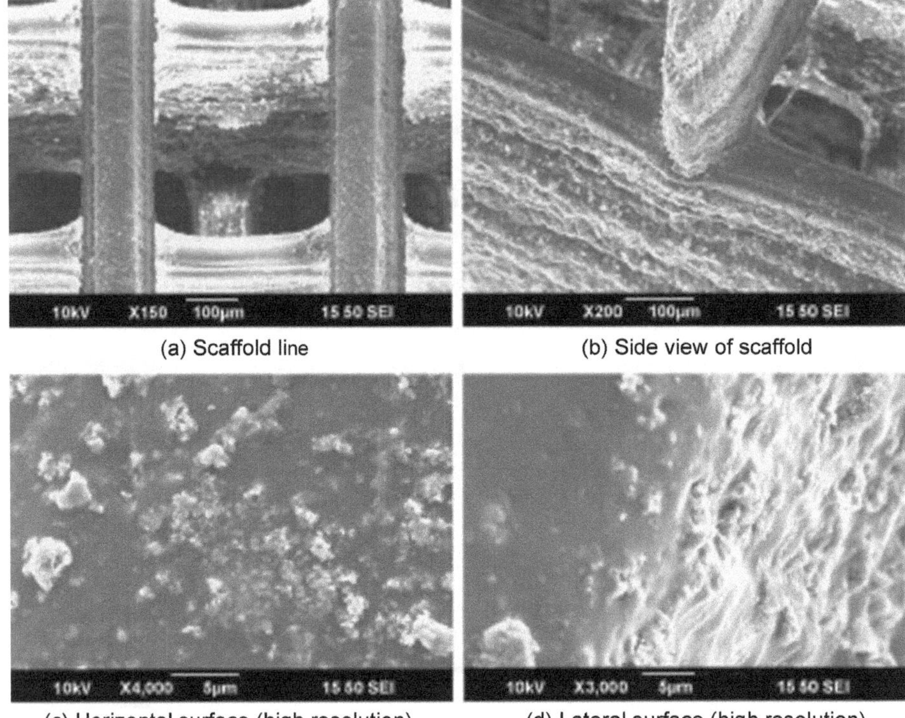

Fig. 16 SEM images of the 3D PPF/DEF scaffolds containing hydroxyapatite [55]

3.2 Polymer/Ceramic Blends

Composite systems, based on polymer and ceramic materials, offer the possibility to produce constructs with increased mechanical properties and bioactivity [71, 87]. To produce polymer-ceramic scaffolds through stereolithography, ceramic particles (hydroxyapatite (HA) and tricalcium phosphate (TCP)) are homogenously dispersed on the polymeric material and subsequently photopolymerized [20, 30, 55, 60]. These scaffolds are usually stiffer and stronger than the polymeric ones, as a result of the incorporation of powder particles. However, the powder not only affects the mechanical properties of the scaffolds, but also increases the viscosity of the polymeric system, affecting the solidification process and the light penetration depth [20, 71].

Lee et al. [55] produced PPF/DEF scaffolds containing 7 % of HA nanopowder, and BAPO as a photoinitiator using the microstereolithography process. MC3T3-E1 pre-osteoblasts, cultured on these scaffolds during 2 weeks, showed better adhesion and proliferation when compared with scaffolds without HA (Fig. 16).

Sharifi et al. [93] produced soft nanocomposite hydrogel structures by the polymerization of a solution, consisting of methacrylate-functionalized triblock copolymers of PEG and PTMC with colloidal dispersions of clay nanoparticles (Laponite

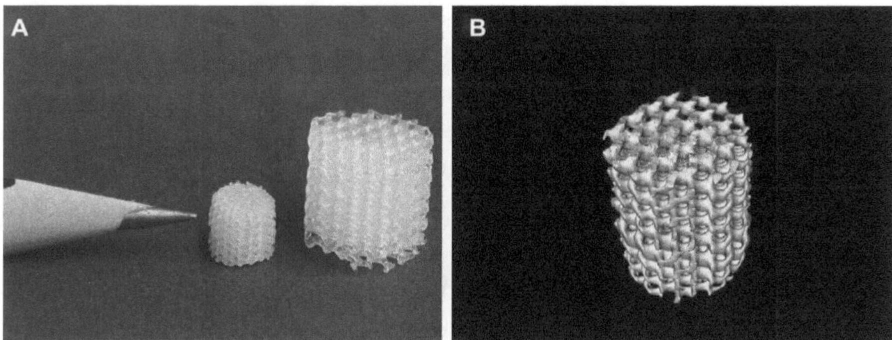

Fig. 17 (A) Macroscopic image of the structures built by stereolithography in the equilibrium water swollen state and after drying. (B) Micro-CT image of the structure in water swollen state [93]

Fig. 18
Stereo-thermal-lithography
system

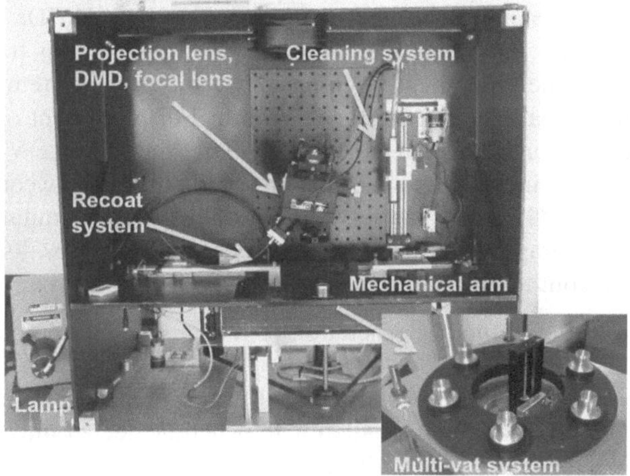

XLG) at different concentrations (2.5 and 5 wt %). Unconfined compression tests were performed regarding the swollen hydrogels, showing that an increasing on the concentration of the Laponite nanoclay improved the compressive modulus. Scaffolds with a gyroid pore network architecture, obtained by stereolithography, showed an interconnected pore network (Fig. 17). In another work, bioactive glass S53P4, an inorganic material with the ability to interact with bone tissue, was combined with a methacrylated PCL polymer to produce porous scaffolds [34]. Bioactive glass was homogeneously distributed through the scaffold and its surface, improving the compression modulus of the construct and the cellular activity of the seeded fibroblasts.

Figure 18 illustrates a mask-based multi-photon and multi-material stereolithographic system. This system, called Stereo-thermal-lithography (STLG), uses a mercury lamp of 350 W as a light source. Appropriated filters split the radiation into two different wavelengths: UV radiation and near-infrared (near-IR) radiation. Optical

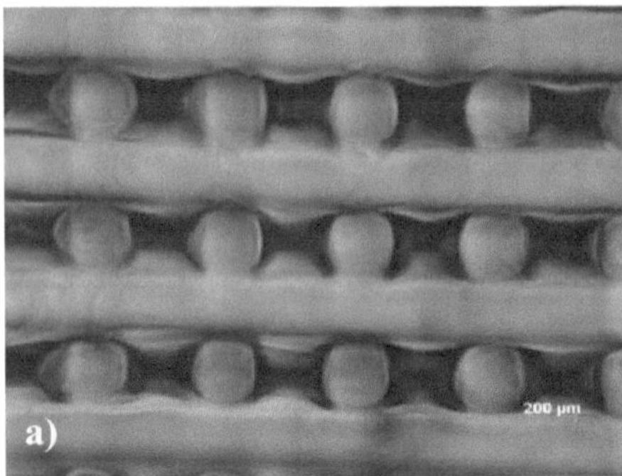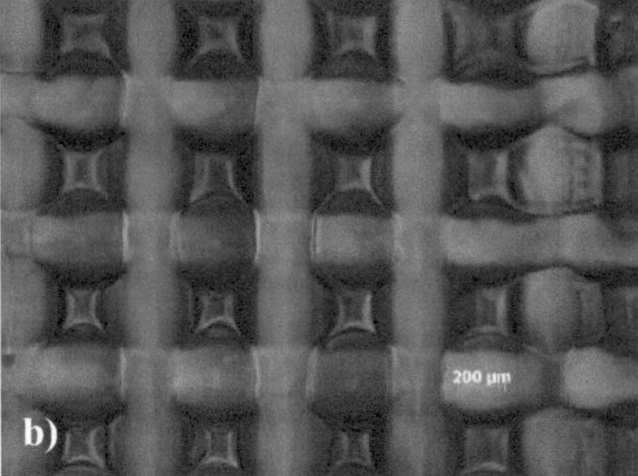

Fig. 19 (**a**) Poly(HEMA) scaffolds containing 2 wt % initiator. (**b**) Poly(HEMA) scaffolds containing 1 wt % initiator

fibres, projection and focal lenses irradiate a UV-DMD and a IR-DMD. A dichroic mirror captures the images projected on both DMDs (1024 × 768 pixels, 14 mm in size), combining them into a single image that is transferred to the liquid polymer. The equipment also includes a multi-vat system enabling the fabrication of multi-material constructs. The vertical displacement of the platform is secured by a positioner uniaxial MYCOSIS® Translation Stage VT-80. This positioner allows vertical increments of 1 μm, at a speed ranging between 0.001 and 20 mm/s.

STLG intends to solve some of the major limitations of conventional stereolithography, such as efficiency, speed and accuracy. Its main advantages over other stereolithographic processes are [10] as follows:

- a more efficient generation of radicals due to the combination of multiple light effects;
- use of small concentrations of the two types of initiator (UV and near-IR initiators), enabling the radiation to penetrate deeper into the polymer;
- a more localized curing reaction, improving the accuracy of the produced models;
- the system has more tunability. Three subsystems can be considered. *Subsystem A*: uses UV radiation to solidify a photopolymer containing a certain amount of UV initiator. *Subsystem B*: uses IR radiation to solidify a photopolymer containing a certain amount of IR initiator. *Subsystem C*: uses both UV and IR radiation to solidify a photopolymer incorporating a certain amount of UV and IR initiators.

The STLG process has been used to produce highly reinforced polymeric systems with metallic and ceramic constructs, PVA and polyHEMA scaffolds (Fig. 19) [33]. The effect of light intensity, photo-initiator concentration, metallic/ceramic powder concentration and powder particle size has been investigated.

Stereolithography has also been used for the direct fabrication of ceramic scaffolds, where the ceramic particles are dispersed on the photocurable polymer and subsequently polymerized. Upon polymerization, the polymer (binder material) is removed using an appropriated thermal or dissolution treatment, and the ceramic particles sintered in order to confer the final properties to the construct [20, 82].

Levy et al. [60] used a ceramic suspension consisting of HA powder and photocurable resin to produce ceramic scaffolds for orbital floor prosthesis. After polymerization, the resin was removed by heating and the resulting ceramic scaffold consolidated by sintering. By combining stereolithography and gel casting, Bian et al. [20] produced an osteochondral beta-tricalcium phosphate/collagen scaffold containing a bone phase with a 3D channel network composed of β-TCP, a cartilage phase consisting of collagen and a transitional interface between the bone and cartilage. Stereolithography was used to produce both bone and transitional phase, through the polymerization of a ceramic suspension. After processing, the binder was removed by pyrolysis, and the porous structure sintered. To produce the cartilage phase, a solution of type-I collagen was casted into a cylindrical mould on the surface of the ceramic scaffold, and then freeze-dried. Finally, the scaffold was immersed into a glutaraldehyde solution (0.5 wt %) to allow the cross-linking of collagen. Bone marrow stromal cells, cultured on the porous scaffolds under perfusion attached well, covering about 60 % of the structure after 7 days.

Ceramic scaffolds can also be obtained through an indirect approach that uses stereolithography to produce lost-moulds, in which ceramic suspensions are casted. The mould is removed by pyrolysis and the scaffold submitted to a sintering process [8]. Chu et al. [30] produced hydroxyapatite scaffolds with two internal architectures (radial and orthogonal design), by casting HA/acrylate suspensions into epoxy moulds created by stereolithography. After polymerization, the epoxy mould and the acrylic binders were removed by sintering, and the scaffolds sintered in a furnace. Scaffolds were implanted in the mandibles of Yucatan minipigs during 5 and 9 weeks. Results showed that the scaffold design has a great influence on the bone regeneration. Scaffolds with a radial design induced the regeneration of new bone tissue as an intact piece at the center of the construct, while the scaffolds with an orthogonal design induced the bone formation as an interpenetrating matrix with the HA implant. A similar approach was used by Kim et al. [49] to produce hydroxyapatite scaffolds, using lost-moulds fabricated by microstereolithography. Recently, Chopra et al. [29] produced glass-ceramic (apatite–mullite glass-ceramic, LG112) scaffolds with simple cubic structure, by gel-casting into moulds produced by stereolithography (Fig. 20a). The moulds were produced by the polymerization of an acrylate polymer and removed prior sintering. Primary human osteoblasts, cultured on the scaffolds composed of only a few slices (Fig. 20b) and square channels of width 400 or 600 µm, showed good adhesion, spreading and proliferation. Despite cells readily proliferate on the scaffold surface, its penetration into the structure was limited, as observed by confocal microscopy (Fig. 20c–e).

4 Final Remarks

Stereolithographic processes have been widely used in tissue engineering for the fabrication of scaffolds for the regeneration of different tissues (e.g. bone, skin, neurons), due to its accuracy, precision, resolution and ability to process a large

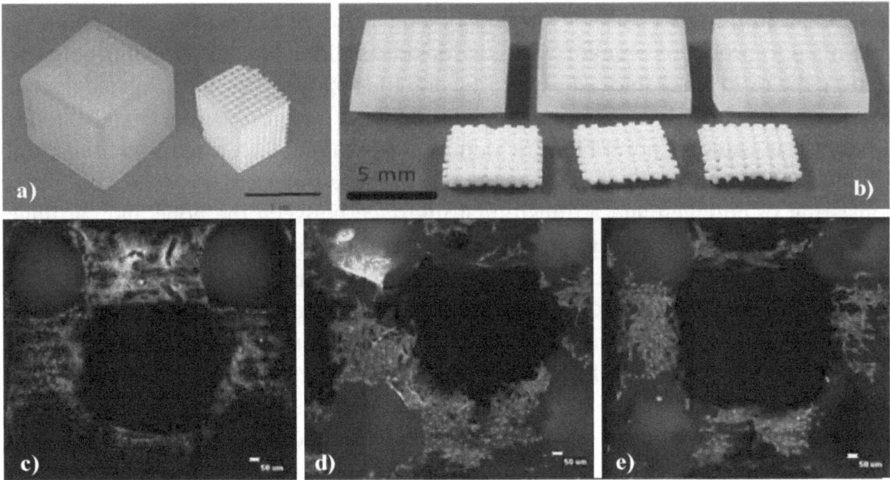

Fig. 20 (**a**) Mould built by stereolithography and respective sintered glass-ceramic scaffold obtained by gel-casting. (**b**) Scaffolds used in the cell culture studies. Confocal fluorescence micrographs of osteoblasts, stained with FITC-conjugated phalloidin for f-actin and DAPI for nuclei on the *top* (**c**), *middle* (**d**) and *bottom* (**e**) of the scaffold, with square channels of with 400 μm [29]

variety of polymer and ceramic materials at physiological temperatures in the presence of cells and growth factors. In spite of current advances, there is a need to produce photocurable systems exhibiting appropriate biocompatibility, biodegradability and cellular interaction to allow the fabrication of scaffolds mimicking the natural ECM constitution and organization. Recent works showed the ability of stereolithography to produce 3D environments for studying the interactions between different cell types, and induce the cell alignment. However, the fabrication of clinically relevant 3D constructs incorporating different cell types in an organized manner is still a great challenge. In order to improve the clinical application of tissue-engineered products obtained by stereolithography, there are relevant challenges to be addressed:

- The development of advanced photocrosslinkable hydrogels mimicking the ECM constituents, allowing the incorporation of multiple cell types with precise and controlled distribution;
- The heterogeneity of natural tissues requiring the fabrication of multimaterial scaffolds resembling its structural and biological organization, providing an optimal environment for the cell attachment, proliferation, differentiation and growth;
- The development of parallel processing strategies to increase the processing rate of stereolithographic techniques and improve the large-scale production towards clinical applications;
- The fabrication of hydrogel scaffolds incorporating living cells requiring the development of advanced optical imaging techniques, capable to perform analysis within the gels without affecting the cell viability or destroying the gels;

- Today, research works are mainly investigating the effect of stereolithography on the cell adhesion, proliferation and differentiation. There is a need for works on the influence of the processing parameters, such as the light intensity and the exposure time on the phenotype of the cells.

Acknowledgements This work was supported by the Portuguese Foundation for Science and Technology through the projects PTDC/EME-PME/098037/2008 and Pest-OE/EME/UI4044/2011.

References

1. Almeida H, Bártolo PJ (2010) Virtual topological optimisation of scaffolds for rapid prototyping. Med Eng Phys 32:775–782
2. Arcaute K, Mann B, Wicker R (2010) Stereolithography of spatially controlled multi-material bioactive poly(ethylene glycol) scaffolds. Acta Biomater 6:1047–1054
3. Arcaute K, Mann BK, Wicker RB (2006) Stereolithography of three-dimensional bioactive poly(ethylene glycol) constructs with encapsulated cells. Ann Biomed Eng 34:1429–1441
4. Arcaute K, Mann BK, Wicker RB (2011) Practical use of hydrogels in stereolithography for tissue engineering applications. In: Bártolo PJ (ed) Stereolithography: materials, processes and applications. Springer, Berlin, pp 299–331
5. Bae MS, Yang DH, Lee JB, Heo DN, Kwon Y-D, Youn IC, Choi K, Hong JH, Kim GT, Choi YS, Hwang EH, Kwon IK (2011) Photo-cured hyaluronic acid-based hydrogels containing simvastatin as a bone tissue regeneration scaffold. Biomaterials 32:8161–8171
6. Bártolo P, Chua CK (2008) Editorial: celebrating the 70th anniversary of professor Yongnian Yan: a life dedicated to science and technology. Virtual Phys Prototyp 3:189–191
7. Bartolo P, Domingos M, Gloria A, Ciurana J (2011) BioCell printing: integrated automated assembly system for tissue engineering constructs. CIRP Ann 60:271–274
8. Bartolo P, Kruth JP, Silva J, Levy G, Malshe A, Rajurkar K, Mitsuishi M, Ciurana J, Leu M (2012) Biomedical production of implants by additive electro-chemical and physical processes. CIRP Ann 61:635–655
9. Bártolo P, Mendes A, Jardini A (2004) Bio-prototyping. In: Collins MW, Brebbia CA (eds) Design and nature II. WIT Press, Ashurst, pp 535–543
10. Bártolo PJ (2001) Optical approaches to macroscopic and microscopic engineering. PhD thesis, University of Reading, UK
11. Bártolo PJ (2006) State of the art of solid freeform fabrication for soft and hard tissue engineering. In: Design and nature III: comparing design in nature with science and engineering, pp 233–243
12. Bartolo PJ (2007) Photo-curing modeling: direct irradiation. Int J Adv Manuf Technol 32:480–491
13. Bartolo PJ (2011) Stereolithographic processes. In: Bartolo PJ (ed) Stereolithography: materials, processes and applications. Springer, Berlin, pp 1–36
14. Bartolo PJ, Chua CK, Almeida HA, Chou SM, Lim ASC (2009) Biomanufacturing for tissue engineering: present and future trends. Virtual Phys Prototyp 4:203–216
15. Bártolo PJ, Domingos M, Patrício T, Cometa S, Mironov V (2011) Biofabrication strategies for tissue engineering. In: Fernandes PR, Bartolo PJ (eds) Advances on modeling in tissue engineering. Springer, Berlin, pp 137–176
16. Bartolo PJ, Gaspar J (2008) Metal filled resin for stereolithography metal part. CIRP Ann 57:235–238
17. Bartolo PJ, Mitchell G (2003) Stereo-thermal-lithography: a new principle for rapid prototyping. Rapid Prototyping J 9:150–156
18. Bártolo PJS, Almeida H, Laoui T (2009) Rapid prototyping and manufacturing for tissue engineering scaffolds. Int J Comput Appl Technol 36:1–9

19. Basu S, Cunningham LP, Pins GD, Bush KA, Taboada R, Howell AR, Wang J, Campagnola PJ (2005) Multiphoton excited fabrication of collagen matrixes cross-linked by a modified benzophenone dimer: bioactivity and enzymatic degradation. Biomacromolecules 6:1465–1474

20. Bian W, Li D, Lian Q, Li X, Zhang W, Wang K, Jin Z (2012) Fabrication of a bio-inspired beta-tricalcium phosphate/collagen scaffold based on ceramic stereolithography and gel casting for osteochondral tissue engineering. Rapid Prototyping J 18:68–80

21. Boucard N, Viton C, Agay D, Mari E, Roger T, Chancerelle Y, Domard A (2007) The use of physical hydrogels of chitosan for skin regeneration following third-degree burns. Biomaterials 28:3478–3488

22. Bryant SJ, Anseth KS (2001) The effects of scaffold thickness on tissue engineered cartilage in photocrosslinked poly(ethylene oxide) hydrogels. Biomaterials 22:619–626

23. Chan V, Collens MB, Jeong JH, Park K, Kong H, Bashir R (2012) Directed cell growth and alignment on protein-patterned 3D hydrogels with stereolithography. Virtual Phys Prototyp 7:219–228

24. Chan V, Zorlutuna P, Jeong JH, Kong H, Bashir R (2010) Three-dimensional photopatterning of hydrogels using stereolithography for long-term cell encapsulation. Lab Chip 10:2062–2070

25. Chang CC, Boland ED, Williams SK, Hoying JB (2011) Direct-write bioprinting three-dimensional biohybrid systems for future regenerative therapies. J Biomed Mater Res, Part B, Appl Biomater 98:160–170

26. Chartier T, Badev A, Abouliatim Y, Lebaudy P, Lecamp L (2012) Stereolithography process: influence of the rheology of silica suspensions and of the medium on polymerization kinetics—Cured depth and width. J Eur Ceram Soc 32:1625–1634

27. Choi J-W, Wicker R, Lee S-H, Choi K-H, Ha C-S, Chung I (2009) Fabrication of 3D biocompatible/biodegradable micro-scaffolds using dynamic mask projection microstereolithography. J Mater Process Technol 209:5494–5503

28. Chong EJ, Phan TT, Lim IJ, Zhang YZ, Bay BH, Ramakrishna S, Lim CT (2007) Evaluation of electrospun PCL/gelatin nanofibrous scaffold for wound healing and layered dermal reconstitution. Acta Biomater 3:321–330

29. Chopra K, Mummery PM, Derby B, Gough JE (2012) Gel-cast glass-ceramic tissue scaffolds of controlled architecture produced via stereolithography of moulds. Biofabrication 4:045002

30. Chu T-MG, Orton DG, Hollister SJ, Feinberg SE, Halloran JW (2002) Mechanical and in vivo performance of hydroxyapatite implants with controlled architectures. Biomaterials 23:1283–1293

31. Claeyssens F, Hasan EA, Gaidukeviciute A, Achilleos DS, Ranella A, Reinhardt C, Ovsianikov A, Shizhou X, Fotakis C, Vamvakaki M, Chichkov BN, Farsari M (2009) Three-dimensional biodegradable structures fabricated by two-photon polymerization. Langmuir 25:3219–3322

32. Cukierman E, Pankov R, Yamada KM (2002) Cell interactions with three-dimensional matrices. Curr Opin Cell Biol 14:633–639

33. Domingos MA, Amalvy JI, Oliveira LM, Pinto EM, Almeida HA, Bartolo PJ (2011) Biofabrication of poly(HEMA) scaffolds through stereolithography. In: Fernandes PR et al (eds) ECCOMAS—international conference on tissue engineering. IST Press, Lisbon

34. Elomaa L, Kokkari A, Närhi T, Seppälä JV (2013) Porous 3D modeled scaffolds of bioactive glass and photocrosslinkable poly(e-caprolactone) by stereolithography. Compos Sci Technol 74:99–106

35. Elomaa L, Teixeira S, Hakala R, Korhonen H, Grijpma DW, Seppälä JV (2011) Preparation of poly(ε-caprolactone)-based tissue engineering scaffolds by stereolithography. Acta Biomater 7:3850–3856

36. García AJ (2005) Get a grip: integrins in cell–biomaterial interactions. Biomaterials 26:7525–7529

37. Garlotta D (2001) A literature review of poly(lactic acid). J Polym Environ 9:63–84

38. Gauvin R, Chen Y-C, Lee JW, Soman P, Zorlutuna P, Nichol JW, Bae H, Chen S, Khademhosseini A (2012) Microfabrication of complex porous tissue engineering scaffolds using 3D projection stereolithography. Biomaterials 33:3824–3834
39. Gittard SD, Ovsianikov A, Akar H, Chichkov B, Monteiro-Riviere NA, Stafslien S, Chisholm B, Shin C-C, Shih C-M, Lin S-J, Su Y-Y, Narayan RJ (2010) Two photon polymerization-micromolding of polyethylene glycol-gentamicin sulfate microneedles. Adv Eng Mater 12:B77–B82
40. Goddard JM, Hotchkiss JH (2007) Polymer surface modification for the attachment of bioactive compounds. Prog Polym Sci 32:698–725
41. Gong Y, Zhou Q, Gao C, Shen J (2007) In vitro and in vivo degradability and cytocompatibility of poly(l-lactic acid) scaffold fabricated by a gelatin particle leaching method. Acta Biomater 3:531–540
42. Huang S, Fu X (2010) Naturally derived materials-based cell and drug delivery systems in skin regeneration. J Control Release 142:149–159
43. Jagur-Grodzinski J (2010) Polymeric gels and hydrogels for biomedical and pharmaceutical applications. Polym Adv Technol 21:27–47
44. Jansen J, Melchels FPW, Grijpma DW, Feijen J (2009) Fumaric acid monoethyl ester-functionalized poly(D,L-lactide)/N-vinyl-2-pyrrolidone resins for the preparation of tissue engineering scaffolds by stereolithography. Biomacromolecules 10:214–220
45. Jeon O, Bouhadir KH, Mansour JM, Alsberg E (2009) Photocrosslinked alginate hydrogels with tunable biodegradation rates and mechanical properties. Biomaterials 30:2724–2734
46. Ji C, Annabi N, Hosseinkhani M, Sivaloganathan S, Dehghani F (2012) Fabrication of poly-DL-lactide/polyethylene glycol scaffolds using the gas foaming technique. Acta Biomater 8:570–578
47. Jung Y, Park MS, Lee JW, Kim YH, Kim S-H, Kim SH (2008) Cartilage regeneration with highly-elastic three-dimensional scaffolds prepared from biodegradable poly(l-lactide-co-ε-caprolactone). Biomaterials 29:4630–4636
48. Kim JM, Park J-J, Lee H-J, Kim W-S, Muramatsu H, Chang S-M (2010) Development of glucose sensor using two-photon adsorbed photopolymerization. Bioprocess Biosyst Eng 33:47–53
49. Kim JY, Lee JW, Lee S-J, Park EK, Kim S-Y, Cho D-W (2007) Development of a bone scaffold using HA nanopowder and micro-stereolithography technology. Microelectron Eng 84:1762–1765
50. Kim K, Dean D, Wallace J, Breithaupt R, Mikos AG, Fisher JP (2011) The influence of stereolithographic scaffold architecture and composition on osteogenic signal expression with rat bone marrow stromal cells. Biomaterials 32:3750–3763
51. Kolambkar YM, Dupont KM, Boerckel JD, Huebsch N, Mooney DJ, Hutmacher DW, Guldberg RE (2011) An alginate-based hybrid system for growth factor delivery in the functional repair of large bone defects. Biomaterials 32:65–74
52. Koroleva A, Gill AA, Ortega I, Haycock JW, Schlie S, Gittard SD, Chichkov BN, Claeyssens F (2012) Two-photon polymerization-generated and micromolding-replicated 3D scaffolds for peripheral neural tissue engineering applications. Biofabrication 4:025005
53. Koskela JE, Turunen S, Ylä-Outinen L, Narkilahti S, Kellomäki M (2012) Two-photon microfabrication of poly(ethylene glycol) diacrylate and a novel biodegradable photopolymer-comparison of processability for biomedical applications. Polym Adv Technol 23:992–1001
54. Lan PX, Lee JW, Seol Y-J, Cho D-W (2009) Development of 3D PPF/DEF scaffolds using micro-stereolithography and surface modification. J Mater Sci, Mater Med 20:271–279
55. Lee JW, Ahn GS, Kim DS, Cho D-W (2009) Development of nano- and microscale composite 3D scaffolds using PPF/DEF-HA and micro-stereolithography. Microelectron Eng 86:1465–1467
56. Lee JW, Kang KS, Lee SH, Kim J-Y, Lee B-K, Cho D-W (2011) Bone regeneration using a microstereolithography-produced customized poly(propylene fumarate)/diethyl fumarate photopolymer 3D scaffold incorporating BMP-2 loaded PLGA microspheres. Biomaterials 32:744–752

57. Lee JW, Lan PX, Kim B, Lim G, Cho D-W (2008) Fabrication and characteristic analysis of a poly(propylenefumarate) scaffold using micro-stereolithography technology. J Biomed Mater Res, Part B, Appl Biomater 87B:1–9

58. Lee K-W, Wang S, Fox BC, Ritman EL, Yaszemski MJ, Lu L (2007) Poly(propylene fumarate) bone tissue engineering scaffold fabrication using stereolithography: effects of resin formulations and laser parameters. Biomacromolecules 8:1077–1084

59. Lee KY, Mooney DJ (2012) Alginate: properties and biomedical applications. Prog Polym Sci 37:106–126

60. Levy RA, Chu T-MG, Halloran JW, Feinberg SE, Hollister S (1997) CT-generated porous hydroxyapatite orbital floor prosthesis as a prototype bioimplant. Am J Neuroradiol 18:1522–1525

61. Lin H, Zhang D, Alexander PG, Yang G, Tan J, Cheng AW-M, Tuan RS (2013) Application of visible light-based projection stereolithography for live cell-scaffold fabrication with designed architecture. Biomaterials 34:331–339

62. Liu VA, Bhatia SN (2002) Three-dimensional patterning of hydrogels containing living cells. Biomed Microdevices 4:257–266

63. Lu Y, Mapili G, Suhali G, Chen S, Roy K (2006) A digital micro-mirror device-based system for the microfabrication of complex, spatially patterned tissue engineering scaffolds. J Biomed Mater Res, Part A 77A:396–405

64. Mapili G, Lu Y, Chen S, Roy K (2005) Laser-layered microfabrication of spatially patterned functionalized tissue-engineering scaffolds. J Biomed Mater Res, Part B, Appl Biomater 75B:414–424

65. Matias JM, Bartolo PJ, Pontes AV (2009) Modelling and simulation of photo-fabrication processes using unsaturated polyester resins. J Appl Polym Sci 114:3673–3685

66. Matsuda T, Mizutani M (2002) Liquid acrylate-endcapped biodegradable poly(ε-caprolactone-co-trimethylene carbonate). II. Computer-aided stereolithographic microarchitectural surface photoconstructs. J Biomed Mater Res 62:395–403

67. Matsuda T, Mizutani M, Arnold SC (2000) Molecular design of photocurable liquid biodegradable copolymers. 1. Synthesis and photocuring characteristics. Macromolecules 33:795–800

68. Melchels FPW, Barradas AMC, van Blitterswijk CA, de Boer J, Feijen J, Grijpma DW (2010) Effects of the architecture of tissue engineering scaffolds on cell seeding and culturing. Acta Biomater 6:4208–4217

69. Melchels FPW, Domingos MAN, Klein TJ, Malda J, Bártolo PJ, Hutmacher DW (2012) Additive manufacturing of tissues and organs. Prog Polym Sci 37:1079–1104

70. Melchels FPW, Feijen J, Grijpma DW (2009) A poly(d,l-lactide) resin for the preparation of tissue engineering scaffolds by stereolithography. Biomaterials 30:3801–3809

71. Melchels FPW, Feijen J, Grijpma DW (2010) A review on stereolithography and its applications in biomedical engineering. Biomaterials 31:6121–6130

72. Meyer W, Engelhardt S, Novosel E, Elling B, Wegener M, Krüger H (2012) Soft polymers for building up small and smallest blood supplying systems by stereolithography. J Funct Biomater 3:257–268

73. Mironov V, Visconti RP, Kasyanov V, Forgacs G, Drake CJ, Markwald RR (2009) Organ printing: tissue spheroids as building blocks. Biomaterials 30:2164–2174

74. Narayan RJ, Doraiswamy A, Chrisey DB, Chichkov BN (2010) Medical prototyping using two photon polymerization. Mater Today 13:42–48

75. Nichol JW, Khademhosseini A (2009) Modular tissue engineering: engineering biological tissues from the bottom up. Soft Matter 5:1312–1319

76. Nichol JW, Koshy ST, Bae H, Hwang CM, Yamanlar S, Khademhosseini A (2010) Cell-laden microengineered gelatin methacrylate hydrogels. Biomaterials 31:5536–5544

77. Oh SH, Park SC, Kim HK, Koh YJ, Lee J-H, Lee MC, Lee JH (2011) Degradation behavior of 3D porous polydioxanone-b-polycaprolactone scaffolds fabricated using the melt-molding particulate-leaching method. J Biomater Sci, Polym Ed 22:225–237

78. Ott HC, Matthiesen TS, Goh S-K, Black LD, Kren SM, Netoff TI, Taylor DA (2008) Perfusion-decellularized matrix: using nature's platform to engineer a bioartificial heart. Nat Med 14:213–221

79. Ovsianikov A, Deiwick A, Van Vlierberghe S, Dubruel P, Möller L, Dräger G, Chichkov B (2011) Laser fabrication of three-dimensional CAD scaffolds from photosensitive gelatin for applications in tissue engineering. Biomacromolecules 12:851–858

80. Ovsianikov A, Malinauskas M, Schlie S, Chichkov B, Gittard S, Narayan R, Löbler M, Sternberg K, Schmitz K-P, Haverich A (2011) Three-dimensional laser micro- and nano-structuring of acrylated poly(ethylene glycol) materials and evaluation of their cytoxicity for tissue engineering applications. Acta Biomater 7:967–974

81. Ovsianikov A, Gruene M, Pflaum M, Koch L, Maiorana F, Wilhelmi M, Haverich A, Chichkov B (2010) Laser printing of cells into 3D scaffolds. Biofabrication 2:014104

82. Peltola SM, Melchels FPW, Grijpma DW, Kellomäki M (2008) A review of rapid prototyping techniques for tissue engineering purposes. Ann Med 40:268–280

83. Peng Y-J, Lu Y-T, Liu K-S, Liu S-J, Fan L, Huang W-C (2013) Biodegradable balloon-expandable self-locking polycaprolactone stents as buckling explants for the treatment of retinal detachment: an in vitro and in vivo study. J Biomed Mater Res, Part A 101A:167–175

84. Pereira R, Carvalho A, Vaz DC, Gil MH, Mendes A, Bártolo P (2013) Development of novel alginate based hydrogel films for wound healing applications. Int J Biol Macromol 52:221–230

85. Pereira R, Almeida HA, Bártolo PJ (2013) Biofabrication of hydrogels constructs. In: Coelho JFJ (ed) Drug delivery systems: advanced technologies potentially applicable in personalized treatments, vol 4. Springer, Berlin

86. Pereira R, Tojeira A, Vaz DC, Mendes A, Bártolo P (2011) Preparation and characterization of films based on alginate and aloe vera. Int J Polym Anal Charact 16:449–464

87. Puppi D, Chiellini F, Piras AM, Chiellini E (2010) Polymeric materials for bone and cartilage repair. Prog Polym Sci 35:403–440

88. Rustad KC, Sorkin M, Levi B, Longaker MT, Gurtner GC (2010) Strategies for organ level tissue engineering. Organogenesis 6:151–157

89. Schüller-Ravoo S, Feijen J, Grijpma DW (2011) Preparation of flexible and elastic poly(trimethylene carbonate) structures by stereolithography. Macromol Biosci 11:1662–1671

90. Schuster M, Turecek C, Weigel G, Saf R, Stampfl J, Varga F, Liska R (2009) Gelatin-based photopolymers for bone replacement materials. J Polym Sci, Part A, Polym Chem 47:7078–7089

91. Seck TM, Melchels FPW, Feijen J, Grijpma DW (2010) Designed biodegradable hydrogel structures prepared by stereolithography using poly(ethylene glycol)/poly(d,l-lactide)-based resins. J Control Release 148:34–41

92. Seppälä J, Korhonen H, Hakala R, Malin M (2011) Photocrosslinkable polyesters and poly(esteranhydride)s for biomedical applications. Macromol Biosci 11:1647–1652

93. Sharifi S, Blanquer SBG, van Kooten TG, Grijpma DW (2012) Biodegradable nanocomposite hydrogel structures with enhanced mechanical properties prepared by photo-crosslinking solutions of poly(trimethylene carbonate)–poly(ethylene glycol)–poly(trimethylene carbonate) macromonomers and nanoclay particles. Acta Biomater 8:4233–4243

94. Shin JH, Lee JW, Jung JH, Cho D-W, Lim G (2011) Evaluation of cell proliferation and differentiation on a poly(propylene fumarate) 3D scaffold treated with functional peptides. J Mater Sci 46:5282–5287

95. Sin DC, Miao X, Liu G, Wei F, Chadwick G, Yan C, Friis T (2010) Polyurethane (PU) scaffolds prepared by solvent casting/particulate leaching (SCPL) combined with centrifugation. Mat Sci Eng, Part C 30:78–85

96. Sionkowska A (2011) Current research on the blends of natural and synthetic polymers as new biomaterials: Review. Prog Polym Sci 36:1254–1276

97. Tan H, Chu CR, Payne KA, Marra KG (2009) Injectable in situ forming biodegradable chitosan–hyaluronic acid based hydrogels for cartilage tissue engineering. Biomaterials 30:2499–2506
98. Tomatsu I, Peng K, Kros A (2011) Photoresponsive hydrogels for biomedical applications. Adv Drug Deliv Rev 63:1257–1266
99. Tomihata K, Suzuki M, Oka T, Ikada Y (1998) A new resorbable monofilament suture. Polym Degrad Stab 59:13–18
100. Tomme SR, Storm G, Hennink WE (2008) In situ gelling hydrogels for pharmaceutical and biomedical applications. Int J Pharm 355:1–18
101. Van Vlierberghe S, Dubruel P, Schacht E (2011) Biopolymer-based hydrogels as scaffolds for tissue engineering applications: a review. Biomacromolecules 12:1387–1408
102. Vasita R, Shanmugam K, Katti DS (2008) Improved biomaterials for tissue engineering applications: surface modification of polymers. Curr Top Med Chem 8:341–353
103. Wang F, Li Z, Khan M, Tamama K, Kuppusamy P, Wagner WR, Sen CK, Guan J (2010) Injectable, rapid gelling and highly flexible hydrogel composites as growth factor and cell carriers. Acta Biomater 6:1978–1991
104. Wang Y, Kim U-J, Blasioli DJ, Kim H-J, Kaplan DL (2005) In vitro cartilage tissue engineering with 3D porous aqueous-derived silk scaffolds and mesenchymal stem cells. Biomaterials 26:7082–7094
105. Weiß T, Hildebrand G, Schade R, Liefeith K (2009) Two-photon polymerization for microfabrication of three-dimensional scaffolds for tissue engineering application. Eng Life Sci 9:384–390
106. Wu X, Liu Y, Li X, Wen P, Zhang Y, Long Y, Wang X, Guo Y, Xing F, Gao J (2010) Preparation of aligned porous gelatin scaffolds by unidirectional freeze-drying method. Acta Biomater 6:1167–1177
107. Xiao W, He J, Nichol JW, Wang L, Hutson CB, Wang B, Du Y, Fan H, Khademhosseini A (2011) Synthesis and characterization of photocrosslinkable gelatin and silk fibroin interpenetrating polymer network hydrogels. Acta Biomater 7:2384–2393
108. Yang Y, Zhao J, Zhao Y, Wen L, Yuan X, Fan Y (2008) Formation of porous PLGA scaffolds by a combining method of thermally induced phase separation and porogen leaching. J Appl Polym Sci 109:1232–1241
109. Yeong W-Y, Chua C-K, Leong K-F, Chandrasekaran M (2004) Rapid prototyping in tissue engineering: challenges and potential. Trends Biotechnol 22:643–652
110. Yoshimoto H, Shin YM, Terai H, Vacanti JP (2003) A biodegradable nanofiber scaffold by electrospinning and its potential for bone tissue engineering. Biomaterials 24:2077–2082
111. Yuan D, Lasagni A, Shao P, Das S (2008) Rapid prototyping of microstructured hydrogels via laser direct-write and laser interference photopolymerisation. Virtual Phys Prototyp 3:221–229
112. Zelzer M, Majani R, Bradley JW, Rose FRAJ, Davies MC, Alexander MR (2008) Investigation of cell–surface interactions using chemical gradients formed from plasma polymers. Biomaterials 29:172–184
113. Zhang J-T, Xue Y-N, Gao F-Z, Huang S-W, Zhuo R-X (2008) Preparation of temperature-sensitive poly(N-isopropylacrylamide)/β-cyclodextrin-grafted polyethylenimine hydrogels for drug delivery. J Appl Polym Sci 108:3031–3037
114. Zhou Y, Ma G, Shi S, Yang D, Nie J (2011) Photopolymerized water-soluble chitosan-based hydrogel as potential use in tissue engineering. Int J Biol Macromol 48:408–413
115. Zorlutuna P, Jeong JH, Kong H, Bashir R (2011) Stereolithography-based hydrogel microenvironments to examine cellular interactions. Adv Funct Mater 21:3642–3651